OKANAGAN UNIVERSITY

P9-DVQ-010

WITHDRAWN

DATE DUE

MAY 2 5 1999	
NOV 2 9 1999	
JUL - 4 2000	
FEB - 5	
JAN 2 5 2003	
NOV 1 9 2003	

BRODART   Cat. No. 23-221

Rethinking Depression
Why Current Treatments Fail

Rethinking Depression
Why Current Treatments Fail

Kristina Downing-Orr

Plenum Press • New York and London

Library of Congress Cataloging-in-Publication Data

On file

ISBN 0-306-45940-X

© 1998 Plenum Press, New York
A Division of Plenum Publishing Corporation
233 Spring Street, New York, N.Y. 10013

http://www.plenum.com

10 9 8 7 6 5 4 3 2 1

All rights reserved

No part of this book may be reproduced, stored in a retrieval system, or transmitted in any
form or by any means, electronic, mechanical, photocopying, microfilming, recording, or
otherwise, without written permission from the Publisher

Printed in the United States of America

Preface

As both an academic and professional psychologist, my background is somewhat unique. Most psychologists either opt for the research route, where they study human behavior in the hope of generating insightful theories, or they choose to work clinically with clients and patients.

The problems with these distinct pathways should seem apparent. In their academic role, research psychologists study and generate numerous theories about people, both as individuals and as social beings. However, while their conclusions may provide the basis for therapeutic work, research psychologists are not clinicians. Conversely, clinical psychologists and other therapists are trained principally to work with clients and patients. While many clinicians carry out research projects, their time is mostly spent offering professional help to people. Although both roles serve to advance the science and practice of psychology, researchers in their ivory towers may find their abstract theories and conclusions are inapplicable in the "real world," whereas therapists might discover they work within prescribed treatment frameworks without questioning the limits of these approaches.

Because of my two professional roles, I have aimed to bridge this gap. Here, I have combined my experiences of researching and treating depression with the intentions of improving treatments and of encouraging better communication between the two psychologies.

Kristina Downing-Orr
Oxford, England

Acknowledgments

Many people provided the inspiration for this book, and I will be eternally grateful for all their assistance.

I owe a debt of gratitude to many of the academics in the Oxford University department of experimental psychology whose lectures and informal chats I found particularly informative. Professor Sue Iversen, Jane Mellanby, Peter McLeod, Paul Harris, and Gordon Claridge were particularly inspiring.

I would also like to express my thanks to Joanna Lawrence, my editor, and Nick Thomas for shaping my ideas into this final coherent form.

Finally, this book would not have been possible without the input and experiences of my clients who should continue to remind health care professionals on a regular basis that people's lives don't always fit into neat little theoretical and treatment boxes.

Contents

Part IV   Recommendations for Improving
Diagnosis and Treatment

I

Current Problems in Understanding Depression

1

Introduction

WHY CURRENT TREATMENTS FOR DEPRESSION FAIL

Clinical depression is now recognized as one of the most common mental health disorders plaguing society today. According to an American Psychiatric Association report (1994), up to 3% of men and 9% of women, roughly about 16 million people, in the United States suffer from the symptoms of major depression at any given time. In the United Kingdom estimates are somewhat higher, where 6% of men and 12% of women, upwards of 4 million people, are depressed (Milligan & Clare, 1994). So prevalent is depression among the adult population that 1 in 20 people are currently suffering from the symptoms of a mood disorder (Milligan & Clare, 1994). Furthermore, there is also evidence to suggest that the number of depressed people is on the rise. Since the Second World War, researchers have estimated that there are now ten times as many depressed patients as ever before (for example, see Seligman, 1989a), and it is now accepted that 1 in 5 people will develop depressive illness in their lifetime. It should not be surprising then that mood disorders are often referred to as the "common cold of psychology" and a "psychiatrist's bread and butter."

Although the symptoms of depression can be severe and debilitating and can destroy the quality of a patient's life, it is estimated that up to 90% of depressed patients can be treated effectively through antidepressant medication, psychological intervention treatment, or a combination of the two (Gold, 1995). However, on closer inspection the true claims of the effectiveness of these different treatment strategies must be viewed with some caution. While the advancements in treatments particularly from the newer antidepressant drugs should be a source of encouragement for depressed patients, studies point to some serious problems with these treatments that impair their effectiveness. First, despite the availability of antidepressants, particularly the so-called "wonder" second-generation drugs, it is estimated that only around 20% of depressed patients are receiving treatment (Gold, 1995), suggesting that the vast majority of people with depressive illness are failing to receive any treatment at all. Second, there are problems even for those people who are taking antidepressants. According to a recent conference paper presented at the 1995 International Psychiatric Conference in Venice, suicide rates among the depressed who have been prescribed drugs have actually increased, not decreased as expected, because of insufficient drug dosages (Mendlewicz & Montgomery, 1995). This means that many patients are suffering from the side effects of the drugs without receiving any of the benefits. Third, while suicide may represent an extreme option even among depressed patients, many people with mood disorders continue to suffer often seriously despite medical intervention, usually from the side effects of antidepressant drugs, lack of progress in psychological therapy, and the stigma and shame associated with depressive illness.

The aim of this book is, therefore, to tackle the very important question: Why do current treatments fail? On the surface there are several immediate explanations that spring to mind. In the first instance, although depression is a complex illness with physical, emotional, motivational, and concentration impairments, there is a tendency for mental health professionals to concentrate almost exclusively on the emotional symptoms. As a result of this bias, many depressed patients are blamed for their symptoms and are dismissed as morally inferior and emotionally unstable. As a consequence, depression and the afflicted patients are not taken seriously and this attitude affects the willingness of physicians and therapists to treat the illness. As part of the 1992 Royal College of Psychiatrists' aim to increase public knowledge about depression, they commissioned a study the results of which found that there is a stigma associated with mental illness and that people with psychiatric problems are seen as weak and unstable, even by mental health professionals (Milligan & Clare, 1994). Furthermore, sharing this viewpoint, non-medical health care professionals were not seen to consider depression as a major illness. Social psychologists refer to this bias as the Fundamental Attribution Error, which points to a contradiction between a participator and an observer in explaining the same event, and I would argue that this bias is relevant for health care professionals who treat depression. According to this theory, when something goes wrong, individuals tend to blame the circumstances of the situation, rather than themselves. Conversely, observers tend to blame the individuals. In terms of treating depression, the Fundamental Attribution Error is a likely explanation for the tendency of health care professionals to blame the depressed individual. This unsympathetic attitude among health care professionals should be met with concern, since depression is an illness that runs a high risk of suicide and parasuicidal behavior in the suffered. Furthermore, as a result of this bias, many patients feel stigmatized and guilty about their symptoms, equating depression with mental breakdown and a moral weakness on their part. Because they believe they deserve to suffer—which reflects both a cardinal symptom of depression and the attitudes of the mental health professionals—depressed people often fail to report problems with prescribed treatments to their physician. In fact, many fail to seek help altogether. Finally, another problem that perpetuates this cycle of ineffective treatment stems from the rigid hierarchy in the medical profession, where physicians are rarely challenged. Because of the reverence in which physicians are held, patients, nurses, and other medical and nonmedical staff tend to obey automatically a physician's prescribed course of treatment without challenge. For example, according to one study (U.S. Health Care Financing Administration, 1982, reported in Cialdini, 1982), every day physicians prescribe the wrong drug dose in at least 12% of cases. Furthermore, even when obvious mistakes are made, usually through a simple typographical error on a prescription bottle that changes the treatment entirely, the instructions for treatment no matter how illogical are still carried out unchallenged (Cialdini, 1982). To illustrate this phenomenon, Cialdini reports an amusing case of a patient who sought treatment for an infection in his right ear. When the physician prescribed ear drops for the right ear, this was abbreviated on the prescription pad to "R ear." However, a typographical mistake regarding the directions on the prescription bottle specified "Rear" instead of "R ear." So, the patient, instead of questioning the logistics of this treatment strategy, administered the ear drops to his rear as instructed. Cialdini's reports of patients and their unwillingness to question even the most ludicrous of medical treatments are humorous. However, they still convey the serious and worrying concern that patients rarely challenge their physicians, even when treatments are ineffective or plainly inappropriate.

These explanations point to a catalog of errors in both diagnosing and treating depression and also hint at the massive misinformation and myths that surround depression. So, despite the encouragement of earlier claims about the effectiveness of treatment for depression, it should now be clear that this optimism is premature. It should also be obvious that these three explanations are themselves limited in clarifying problems with treatments for depression and that they beg the further questions as to why treatments for depression fail. Namely:

1. Why are the emotional symptoms of mood disorders, which lead to stigma, emphasized while the physical, motivational, and concentration disturbances associated with depression remain ignored?
2. Recognizing the gravity of the illness and the heightened risk of suicide among sufferers, why is depression stigmatized when other diseases are not?
3. Why are depressed patients seen as morally inferior, emotionally unstable, and sometimes even blamed for their illness while those afflicted with other health problems, such as cancer, AIDS, or injuries resulting from destructive behavior, held less accountable?

In order to demonstrate further the reasons why current treatment strategies for depression fail, questions such as these need to be addressed. With this book, I hope to clarify and explain the problems with treatment strategies and point to two grave errors in the ways in which depression is conceptualized, which in turn affect the ways the illness is diagnosed and treated. First, scientists, researchers, and mental health practitioners erroneously insist on rigidly viewing depression as *either* a psychological illness *or* a biological one. Where biological illnesses are accepted as legitimate because they point to some form of organic malfunction, psychological illnesses tend to be viewed as imaginary and therefore not credible. Furthermore, in emphasizing only these emotional and biological causes of depression, scientists and health care professionals ignore the fact that there could very well be more than one cause of depression and other organic causes that are not currently recognized.

Second, because of this bias toward emotional symptoms, health care professionals often fail to make the preliminary diagnostic distinction between primary depression and secondary depression. That is, they fail to distinguish between depression as an illness in its own right and depressive symptoms that are indicative of another health complaint. In summary, problems in terms of both conceptualizing and diagnosing depression lead not only to stigma, but also to ineffective treatments that fail.

In the course of research, I found evidence that at the heart of the earlier explanations about the problems surrounding treatment effectiveness are the wide-ranging theoretical problems about the nature of depression. Mostly, in evaluating the effectiveness of drug and psychological therapies, there is too much focus on the treatment outcomes themselves. Instead, I suggest that treatment for depression should first be viewed as a process beginning with theories and explanations about the nature of the illness, which then serve as the basis for diagnosing and treating depression, because within this process lies the true reason why treatments are limited in terms of their effectiveness.

The main problems with both drug and many talk therapies stem from a breakdown in the whole of this process. Fundamentally, there is a lack of consensus among researchers and health care professionals in their attempts to explain and define depression, which, in turn, contributes to a breakdown in the ways the illness is diagnosed. With many different, even conflicting, views on defining and explaining the causes of depression, it should not be surprising that diagnostic methods and treatment strategies are also limited. It might seem obvious that the successful outcome of treatments for any illness depends both on a clear understanding among health care professionals of exactly what constitutes the disease and on a conclusive diagnosis that confirms the patient is in fact suffering from the illness in question. However, when it comes to depression, there is a whole range of definitions that are often vague, conflicting, outdated, and lacking in scientific evidence to support their claims. So, in regards to conceptualizing depression, there are clear theoretical problems that need addressing. In terms of diagnosis, health care professionals often shun the use of reliable and objective laboratory tests that would confirm or rule out depressive illness, even though these are readily available. Because diagnosis of depression tends to be subjective and based on patients' own explanations of their symptoms, there is a strong likelihood of diagnostic error. Therefore, even with the advances and breakthroughs evident in recent years in treating depression, particularly with the advent of antidepressant drugs, many patients are misdiagnosed and inevitably receive treatments that are of little use. Figure 1 illustrates this process.

WHY MISINFORMATION ABOUT DEPRESSION ABOUNDS

The question that needs to be addressed is why so much misinformation about depression abounds. The illness is complex and this is obviously the main source of the problem. Most of our professional knowledge on the subject of depression comes from academic research, that is, studies by biochemists, neuroscientists, psychologists, psychiatrists, and other scientists. However, we still know so

Problems in understanding the nature of depression
↓
Problems in diagnosing depression
↓
Problems in treating depression
↓
Problems in evaluating treatments for depressions

Figure 1.   The process of breakdown in treating depression.

little about human physiology and how the brain functions and this lack of knowledge is in many ways just as important to diagnostic and treatment strategies. Old views of the illness are being constantly replaced and updated by breakthroughs and newer discoveries, but this approach to studying depression is still in many ways haphazard and random and scientists are only slowly solving the puzzle of depression. Very little of what researchers and health care professionals know is conclusive, so scientists often make assumptions about the illness that are intuitive and commonsensical. But the exact nature of depression is nevertheless still unknown. What scientists believe to be true about depression today may or may not be so tomorrow. This is particularly important for health care professionals to understand because these current theories are really little more than temporary guidelines that may or may not stand the test of time. However, when accepted as fact, they, in turn, become the basis for treatment.

PART ONE: CURRENT PROBLEMS IN UNDERSTANDING DEPRESSION

This book addresses many of these queries and is divided into four parts. The first part aims to clarify and make sense of the many inconsistencies currently existing in the literature on the origins of the illness and presents for discussion (1) explanations of depression, (2) a client case study that illustrates a patient's problems in trying to obtain effective treatment for her depressed symptoms, (3) evaluations of theories about biological causes, (4) evaluations of theories about psychological causes, and (5) alternative theories.

Basically, in addition to the many, conflicting explanations of the nature of depression, there is the deeply entrenched bias that depression is either an emotional illness or a biological illness caused by brain dysfunction. While there are obviously likely cases of depression that are attributed to either psychological or biological causes alone, this rigid emphasis is outdated and ignores the more current explanation that depression is a psychological illness in which both the mind and the body play important roles. In accepting the psychobiological nature of depression, stigma and blame are automatically reduced and other potential explanations about the causes of this illness can be explored.

More specifically, the chapters in Part One address the following points:

1. There is little consensus about the nature of depression among health care professionals.
2. Health care professionals tend to define and explain depression in a variety of very different, contradictory, and incompatible ways. They tend to focus exclusively either on the physiological causes of depression or on the emotional and ignore the important roles of both the mind and the body.
3. Biological theories tend to focus too narrowly on neurochemical dysfunction.
4. Psychological theories about the nature of depression are often outdated, lack scientific evidence, fail to incorporate more recent findings about the physiological nature of the illness, and make presumptions about human behavior that are not supported by the evidence.
5. Because of their narrow and rigid interpretations about mood disorders, biological and psychological theories about the causes of depression also tend to ignore the hundreds of other neurological, pharmacological, and physiological causes of depression.
6. Current physiological and psychological theories about depression also fail to accept that depression can be a normal reaction to someone's personal circumstances.
7. In determining the causal nature of depression, theories tend to ignore the very real possibility that symptoms can be multicausal even in the same individual.

PART TWO: CURRENT PROBLEMS IN DIAGNOSING DEPRESSION

Part Two explores some of the problems associated with the diagnosis of depression. Because of the current flaws in explaining the nature and origin of depressive illness and because of the rigid viewpoints that depression is caused *either* by a neurochemical breakdown *or* an emotional one, the diagnostic process often tends to be problematic. The main problem with current diagnostic practices stems from the subjective approach physicians and psychologists take. With most illnesses, physicians administer laboratory tests to confirm or rule out disease; however, with depression, the diagnostic process tends not to include objective methods. Furthermore, because emotional symptoms are indicative of other physiological, neurological, and pharmacological health problems, the danger with this practice is that patients are diagnosed and treated for depression—an illness that they may not even have—when the true cause of their symptoms may go undetected. Some of the points to be addressed in the chapters in this section include:

1. Diagnosing depression tends to be subjective and therefore unreliable. Instead of using objective diagnostic tests, physicians and psychologists often diagnose depression based on subjective methods, usually the patients' own self-reports. Because emotional symptoms are often severe with depressive illness and most people will attempt to make sense of their symptoms, physicians and patients may just accept that a personal catastrophe is to blame, even when there is an underlying organic cause.

2. There is a tendency to ignore the wide range of symptom clusters associated with depression. In many cases, because of the emphasis on the emotional symptoms of depression, physicians and health care professionals tend to ignore the many other physical, concentration, and motivational disturbances associated with depression. As a result, many health care professionals fail to detect symptoms of depression and their patients remain undiagnosed.

3. Physicians and nonmedical professionals have a tendency to diagnose on the basis of stereotypes. Women, the elderly, and ethnic minorities are more likely to be diagnosed with depression, because they are viewed by the mainly white, male, middle-class medical establishment as emotionally weaker.

4. Physicians and therapists often too readily diagnose pri-

mary depression and ignore that secondary depression may be to blame. Although depression (primary) is an illness in its own right, symptoms of emotional distress (secondary) can also indicate other health problems.

5. Health care professionals tend to overrely on diagnostic categories, such as the reactive/endogenous classification. These categorical distinctions are outdated and ignore the interaction of the psychobiological nature of the illness.

PART THREE: EVALUATING TREATMENTS FOR DEPRESSION

Part Three looks at problems in treating depression. Recognizing the problems in diagnosing depression, especially the subjective nature of the process, it should not be surprising that treatment strategies are often ineffective and haphazard. Theoretical explanations and the diagnosis of depression remain profoundly influenced by the mind/body distinction and so treatment strategies also fall along these lines. Physiological treatments tend to include antidepressant drugs, although in rare circumstances electroshock therapy is prescribed. Furthermore, sometimes in lieu of drugs and in other instances in combination with them, psychological therapy is also used.

The chapters in Part Three consider some of the more glaring problems with treatment strategies that must be addressed if therapies to combat depression are to be valid, reliable, and effective. These limitations include:

1. Prescribing drug and psychological treatments for patients who are not suffering from depression.
2. Ignoring other possible therapies in favor of those that correct neurochemical or emotional breakdown.
3. Prescribing antidepressant drugs even though the side effects can be severe and health care professionals still do not fully understand their long-term safety.
4. Failure on the part of psychologists and other nonmedical therapists to advise their clients to seek medical attention for their symptoms before they begin therapy.

5. Addressing the limitations of the psychological therapies. Some are outdated, ignore the nature of depression and the needs of the depressed individual, make assumptions about human behavior that are not supported by scientific data, fail to keep up with advances in human physiology, and treat the symptoms rather than the causes of the illness.
6. Recognizing that psychological treatments differ in terms of effectiveness and that some forms of therapy might even be considered dangerous for a depressed patient.

PART FOUR: RECOMMENDATIONS FOR IMPROVING DIAGNOSIS AND TREATMENT

Part Four presents guidelines for improved diagnosis and treatment. In terms of diagnosis, this part presents and identifies some of the laboratory medical tests that can confirm or rule out depression. If depression is confirmed, these medical tests can indicate more clearly the specific type of depressive illness. If depression is ruled out, then physicians can further their investigation to determine the true cause of the emotional symptoms.

In this section, I also offer recommendations and suggestions for treating depression, including personal development, encouraging and motivating clients to take active control of their health care management, dietary considerations, and relaxation exercises.

In summary, treatment strategies for depression so often fail and are ineffective because there is little consensus or uniformity among researchers and health care professionals about the theoretical nature of the illness. These contradictory, conflicting, and inconclusive notions about depression, however, form the basis for diagnosis and treatment. In the following chapters, I present and explain the breakdown in this process. However, it will be more illuminating to demonstrate the problems with the treatment process through a case study example. Such is the focus of Chapter Two.

2

Shelly
A Case Study

To any health care professional working with depressed patients or clients, the discussion introduced in the last chapter should clearly point to the often confusing state of both diagnosing and treating clinical depression. Many questions remain unanswered and despite the continuing breakthroughs, conflicts and misinformation about the nature of depression continue to flourish. This is much more than an academic debate, as individuals with depression so often continue to suffer and in some cases are even denied a cure. And, because depressed patients are at a higher risk for suicide, inadequate or ineffective medical treatment for depression often does mean the difference between life and death. So, rethinking the entire treatment process for depression—from conceptualization to diagnosis to therapy—is essential to improve the quality of patient care and the effectiveness of measures to combat the illness.

Although the basis of this book is a theoretical analysis and discussion, as both an academic and a practitioner, I believe that a client case study best illustrates the current problems in treating depression. Shelly was a 30-year-old American client living in England who had been suffering from depression for a number of years and who had received ineffective antidepressant and psychological treatments.

Shelly remembers very clearly when her mood disorder first developed. And, because most people try to make some sense of their lives when something goes wrong, when Shelly initially began to feel depressed, she believed her symptoms were connected to her recent move to London, where her husband, David, was offered a job working for a bank. Originally, Shelly had been excited by, and was indeed looking forward to her stay in England. Since she and her husband first met as undergraduates, both had expressed an ambition to travel, to see the world, and this opportunity for David to work in London seemed "like a dream come true."

Shortly after their arrival in England, however, Shelly began to sense that something was "not quite right" with her moods. She was "inexplicably sad, but sometimes very anxious." However, she just dismissed these emotional disturbances as adjustment difficulties and homesickness that go along with moving to a new place.

In these early days, Shelly tried to distract her attention from her sadness and anxieties by applying for jobs as an accountant. As she had professional experience in the United States and was highly regarded by her boss, she assumed she would have minimal difficulties finding work in London. However, she was unsuccessful even in getting an interview and the steady stream of rejection letters that she received began damaging her self-esteem, making her moods feel worse. Furthermore, David was spending long hours at the office in order to settle in and make a good impression. When he did return home, usually late in the evening, he was exhausted and would go right to bed.

Without a job and lacking the opportunity to meet new people, Shelly felt isolated in spending so much time on her own. The few social contacts she did have were her husband's work colleagues. When they did go out, David and his co-workers wanted to talk shop most of the time, leaving Shelly feeling excluded, "totally invisible." In fact, Shelly began to resent her husband's lack of attention. "He just didn't seem interested in me any more. Any free time he did have, he wanted to go out with the boys from work and when he was home on weekends, he was just too tired. So much for being honeymooners."

All of these various difficulties began to mount up and although Shelly had always described herself as independent and adventurous, everything seemed to be "getting on top" of her. She began to feel apathetic, bored, isolated, and "not really interested in doing anything." She became irritable, impatient, and used to snap at

David as soon as he came in from the office at night. Her moods were unpredictable; sometimes she would be apathetic and lethargic, and at other times, bad-tempered, angry, and aggressive. So, despite having been married for just a few months, David and Shelly's relationship was becoming strained.

As the weeks and months progressed, Shelly continued to withdraw socially and even when she did force herself to accompany David out to dinner with his co-workers, she felt as though she was just "going through the motions." She didn't enjoy going out, or meeting new people anymore. In fact, she felt resentful that she was forced to make an effort for people who did not really care if she were present or not. As someone who had always enjoyed going to parties and socializing, Shelly began to lose confidence in her ability to meet people. She eventually stopped going out with David. She no longer "had the energy to make the effort."

Some days she wouldn't even get out of bed.

Clearly, Shelly was showing signs of depression and she lived in this state continually for an entire year and intermittently like this for several years. After a few months of Shelly's feeling "unusually despondent," David suggested that she should seek professional help, because he was having difficulties understanding and coping with his wife. At first she resisted his pleas for her to seek professional help, but as her mood swings and anxiety became worse, Shelly eventually agreed to see a physician.

After she made an appointment to see her physician, Shelly began to feel relieved. She assumed that if she sought medical attention, maybe even saw a psychiatrist, she would obtain the information and help that she now realized she needed. Unfortunately, far from helping her to feel better, the physicians and therapists she saw had the effect of making her feel much worse, because of the stigma they imposed on her and their professional arrogance and inability to provide information and guidance. Shelly firmly believes that they even contributed to her mental health problems.

So, where she had sought medical help hoping she would feel better, instead she found physicians who were unsympathetic, patronizing, and superior, who seemed only interested in judging her as some inadequate, emotional woman. The first physician was dismissive of her symptoms and her worries and made her feel that she was nothing more than a "self-indulgent, pathetic whiner who was wasting his time." He spent all of five minutes listening to Shelly describe her symptoms and her concerns about her deteriorating mental health and promptly dismissed her worries stating that adjustment difficulties were normal when moving to a new country. If Shelly did not have the strength and resilience of character to cope with living abroad (which he felt he had to remind her was an opportunity of a lifetime), then clearly she was immature and needed to grow up. Undeterred, but discouraged by the lack of help, Shelly saw other physicians in both the United Kingdom and the United States, but they were all equally unsympathetic and unhelpful. Some even warned her that if she failed to change her negative and pessimistic attitude, David would leave her. Perhaps she should consider having a baby, one physician suggested, as "time was marching on," while another one claimed she was "psychoneurotic," and a third told her she should turn to God.

After each new attempt to seek help from physicians, Shelly's already fragile self-esteem became even more profoundly shattered and she felt even more guilty and personally inadequate because she also felt she was letting her husband down. Shelly knew she was feeling emotionally unstable and was frightened by the severity of her symptoms, and she had gone to these physicians for help. But they had only made her feel even more inadequate, vulnerable, and alone. They had treated Shelly as though she were some sort of oddity, a "freak," because she suffered from depression.

After several attempts to seek help from physicians and the failure of the prescribed antidepressants and tranquilizers, which made her feel "doped up, tired, a zombie," Shelly responded by ceasing to seek medical help altogether—a practice that is dangerous for depressed patients. She decided instead to turn to the "talk" therapists, assuming a counselor or a psychologist would offer more sympathy and teach her how to cope with her moods. However, this was not the case.

The first therapist she saw claimed he was experienced in helping depressed people and their partners cope with the pressures of the illness. He listened patiently to her concerns about her deteriorating mental health, her lack of success in finding a job, and her increasingly strained relationship with her husband. At the end of the session, his only advice was for Shelly "not to make another appointment," because he was concerned she could become "addicted" to therapy. Stunned by his strange response, Shelly left his office without asking him what he meant.

Shelly's later experiences with other therapists were no more beneficial or supportive. Many were unresponsive, cold, and unfeeling. They also treated her as though she were a weak, inadequate female, unable to handle her emotions.

> They kept asking me, probing me about my relationship with my parents, which was fine. My parents had their ups and downs and were very different people. They sometimes argued, and they weren't exactly the most demonstrative of people. Sure, I would describe my parents as cold, but mine was certainly not the dysfunctional home my therapists were trying to portray. I love my parents.
>
> But all these people I saw, you know, they kept harping on and on about my parents. They kept telling me I was depressed because I felt abandoned by my husband in a new country just as I had felt abandoned by my parents. At first I believed them, after all they are the professionals, they should know, but I still didn't get any better.

Shelly's experiences with physicians and therapists left her feeling confused and her attempts to seek professional help and relief from her symptoms were fruitless, for many of the reasons expressed in the Introduction. Shelly was diagnosed on the basis of a stereotype, by both male and female mental health professionals, and on the basis of her own subjective explanations about why she thought she was depressed. Furthermore, far from helping her, Shelly's physicians and therapists were essentially unresponsive.

As a therapist, I was amazed by Shelly's experiences with health care professionals, but they are certainly not unique. Most depressed individuals who come to me for treatment relate similar stories about their previous attempts to seek help.

Eventually, Shelly was referred to me and soon began receiving the information, the direction, and the medical and psychological advice that had previously been sorely lacking. The most important discovery for her recovery was showing her that symptoms of depression should never be accepted at face value and in fact can also be dangerous if they are. Granted, her life was certainly troublesome for a few years and on the surface it seems understandable to assume that her depressive symptoms were caused by her adjustment difficulties and homesickness, which were exacerbated by her inability to find a job and the social isolation she faced. However, because depression manifests itself through both psychological and physical symptoms, even if the cause is a biochemical malfunction, an individual's sense of emotional well-being is also likely to be impaired.

Shelly's own experiences demonstrated most profoundly the interaction between emotional and physical symptoms. Because she felt so physically unwell, everything else in her life also seemed pretty hopeless—her present, her past, her future. And she then began to attribute her depressive symptoms to external factors and the difficulties she was facing adjusting to life abroad, because she just *assumed* they must be the cause. However, if any of the physicians had explored her symptoms further, if they had thoroughly examined Shelly and administered laboratory tests, they might have learned, as we later discovered, that the most severe symptoms, especially the mood swings and anxiety attacks, were not caused by depression at all, but rather by her intolerance to sugar.

In the course of our therapy, Shelly had discovered that it was her sweet tooth, the chocolates, cakes and cookies, and other comfort foods that she was eating that were causing her mood swings. Why she should have developed those symptoms at that time in her life remains a mystery. Furthermore, particularly at times when she both fed her sweet tooth and drank coffee, Shelly would become anxious, irritable, and panicky and develop more severely the highs and then the crashing lows that typified her mood swings. However, once she eliminated sugar from her diet and reduced her caffeine intake, her moods immediately improved and the worst symptoms of her depression disappeared. Ironically, a recent study has found that women who drink at least two cups of coffee a day seem less likely to develop depression, but Shelly still has to be careful with her caffeine intake—something I advise all of my clients to regulate.

Shelly's example also highlights the importance of understanding that depressive illness can have more than one cause. In addition to the coffee and sugar intolerance, Shelly also began to suffer for the first time from symptoms of seasonal affective disorder (SAD). She first noticed her mood disturbances in October, the month of her arrival in England. So, in addition to her problems with caffeine and sugar intake, the changing seasons also caused her illness. Shelly still suffers from seasonal affective disorder, the symptoms of which normally begin for her at the end of August and ease up in February. But at least now she knows to expect these symptoms at the end of the summer and she knows what they are, so she is no longer afraid when they first appear.

Learning to interpret Shelly's symptoms and monitoring her moods eventually helped us to discover the causes of her symptoms, enabling her to cope with her illness and then, finally, to recover. Although the process was long and sometimes frustrating, Shelly is now emotionally strong and stable. So it is essential that symptoms of depression are never accepted at face value and a thorough medical examination, using the *appropriate diagnostic tests,* must be offered to every patient who complains of depression. Psychologists, counselors, and other non-medically trained health care professionals must also insist that their clients first be examined by a physician before they begin their own psychological treatments. This is the only conclusive way to begin isolating the cause of the illness and to provide effective treatment.

Shelly's case illustrates some of the many current problems with the ways depression is understood, diagnosed, and treated. The physicians and therapists obviously believed that she was to blame for her symptoms and her failure to improve and because guilt is one of the cardinal symptoms of depression, Shelly's sense of her own inadequacy was magnified by their attitudes. The physicians prescribed tranquilizers, which Shelly did not want to take, and the therapists were looking for explanations for the cause of her symptoms, which proved not to be relevant. In neither case was Shelly offered practical help and solutions that would lead to effective treatment, let alone a cure. So, for improved treatment, a true understanding of the nature and origins of depressive illness must be explored.

3

Toward a More Definitive Understanding of Depression

Shelly's experiences in attempting to seek help for depression point to the inadequacies in the ways many physicians and other health care professionals conceive, diagnose, and treat depression. At the heart of the problem often seems to be a lack of accurate, updated information about the nature of depression, which in turn leads to a breakdown in the diagnostic and treatment processes.

The aim of this chapter is to offer a much clearer understanding of the nature of depression. The present lack of reliable information about depression breeds both ignorance and stigma, even among mental health professionals. Therefore, in order to provide a basis for effective and reliable diagnosis and treatment, it is first necessary to offer a more accurate and factual definition of depression.

This chapter attempts this challenge, by first presenting and clarifying some of the more pervasive myths about depression. Then, I present some of the many widespread definitions of depression currently used by researchers and health care professionals to explain the illness and also offer an alternative definition taking into account more recent scientific breakthroughs about the illness. Finally, in order to further understand the nature of the illness, it is also important to be able to distinguish clinical depression from a temporary low mood state. This clarification is also essential because the word *depression* is bandied about in common parlance. Since most people feel down or sad at certain times in their lives, they often mistakenly assume that these temporary low mood states are synonymous with depression. Because stigma about the illness abounds and because evidence has been described in the Introduction to show that many health care professionals fail to acknowledge the serious suffering associated with depression, the ability to distinguish between the common everyday understanding of normal sadness and a clinical illness is important for diagnosis and treatment.

CHALLENGING THE MYTHS ABOUT DEPRESSION

I will first attempt my goal of clarifying the nature of depression by demonstrating what depression is not. Presenting and challenging some of the more deeply entrenched myths about mood disorders is important in this process because they are so widespread and have become accepted as facts, in turn influencing the effectiveness of diagnosis and treatment, in addition to breeding stigma, fear, and shame.

Myth No. 1: Depression is the result of a character flaw or moral weakness.

Despite the pervasive belief held by many health care professionals that depression is the result of a person's inability to cope with his or her problems, current research findings stress that mood disorders should be viewed as a psychobiological illness, that is, a biological problem that expresses itself in part through emotional symptoms.

Myth No. 2: Symptoms of depression should not be taken as seriously as other major health problems like cancer or heart disease.

Severe mood disturbances leave people more susceptible to suicide so their symptoms should be taken very seriously. Unfortunately, while cancer and heart disease patients receive sympathy, support, and medical assistance, because of the myths surrounding mood disturbances, depressed individuals often do not or are made to feel they do not deserve help.

Myth No. 3: All emotional symptoms point to depression.

Many health complaints, some minor, some life threatening, have emotional symptoms associated with them. So an accurate diagnosis to conclusively confirm or rule out depression is essential for effective and correct treatment.

Myth No. 4: All the depressed person has to do is to stop wallowing in self-pity and adopt a more positive attitude in order to feel better.

Depression is not a problem of attitude or outlook. It is an illness that requires medical attention. There is a wide range of effective treatments available, including antidepressants, ECT, and different approaches to therapy.

Myth No. 5: Depression is either an emotional disorder or an illness caused by a neurochemical imbalance.

Depression should be seen as a psychobiological illness, in which the mind and body are affected. Since people try to make sense of their symptoms when they are feeling down, there is a tendency for people to try to explain their mood disturbances in terms of their current difficulties. Because depressed people filter their thoughts, memories, and perceptions of themselves through a veil of negativity—a standard characteristic of the illness whatever the true cause of the symptoms—health care professionals should be more willing to see beyond their clients' seemingly commonsensical and accurate explanations of their symptoms. As Shelly's example demonstrated, even when a client's life appears to be turbulent and distressing, practitioners must not automatically assume that the individual's personal situation is the cause of the illness.

DEFINING DEPRESSION

These myths about the nature of depression need to be addressed and clarified if clients and patients are to receive the best possible support and care. The pervasiveness of these myths and their widespread acceptance among mental health professionals therefore need to be challenged and discussed.

One important way to combat these myths and destigmatize

depression is through information. However, explaining and defining depression is not an easy task. Despite its common usage in everyday language, the word *depression* is not easily defined. In fact, the Royal College of Psychiatrists launched a campaign in 1992 (Milligan & Clare, 1994) designed to increase the public's understanding of depression and found that most people had great difficulty in defining the term.

The inability among members of the public polled in this study to explain depression is understandable. The illness is complex, and academics, researchers, biochemists, and others admit that they still do not know enough about the illness. A typical working definition usually falls along the lines of:

Depression is a psychological disorder characterized by long bouts of severe mood disturbance or excessive elation, which are unconnected with the individual's present situation.

However, for all kinds of reasons, this definition is limited and provides a breeding ground for ignorance. First, this definition wrongly emphasizes that depression is a psychological illness and ignores the psychobiological nature of the disease. Again, emotional symptoms do not automatically mean a psychiatric disorder. Second, by focusing on the psychological nature of the illness, definitions such as these ignore the other cardinal symptoms of depression including physiological, motivational, and concentration disturbances. Third, a definition such as this one ignores the complex nature of the illness. Another problem with this definition is its ambiguity; it might serve to describe in vague, general terms some aspect of a particular type of depression, but it falls short of explaining what depression is.

If this definition is too broad, working definitions for scientists and health care professionals tend to be too narrow and rigid. The biggest problem in terms of defining depression is the lack of consensus about the nature of the illness, which stems primarily from the many diverse, conflicting, and confusing explanations that exist. For example, to one group of professionals, depression is the result of hidden and unresolved childhood traumas; to a second group, it is a malfunction of brain chemistry; to a third group, it is the result of poor social skills; and to a fourth group, certain individuals are regarded to be prone to depression because of irrational, negative thinking and highly critical self-appraisals. Feelings of helplessness or hopelessness seem to be the central causes for other professionals. It is evident, then, that there are many, very different, explanations for the causes of depression, which flourish in academic journals in the form of unresolved theoretical disputes. The main problems with these definitions stem first from the fact that they are based on the erroneous assumption that depression is *either* emotional *or* biological in nature. Second, they tend more to describe the symptoms of depression and fail to offer any valid explanations about the illness. Third, these definitions tend to be fractured, contradictory, and conflicting and indicate a lack of consensus among researchers and health care professionals about the nature of the illness. As a result, instead of offering a clarification about depression, understanding and explaining the illness automatically becomes rife with ambiguities.

How Should Depression Be Defined?

In my view, any credible and valid definition of depression must first address the complex nature of the illness and must indicate that depression is at once a disease and a symptom of another health problem and that the illness has a wide range of symptoms and causes. Most likely, depression comprises many different illnesses and any definition must reflect this. Second, definitions of depression must now challenge the erroneous assumption that the illness is caused by either psychological or physiological factors alone. In this way, I would suggest and stress that the illness is psychobiological in nature—a physical illness with a whole range of symptoms including emotional, motivational, and concentration disturbances. In other words, depression is an illness, several illnesses, or symptomatic of another health problem that strikes both the mind and the body. While this definition might itself be open to charges of ambiguity, my intention is first to broaden the currently held rigid views about the nature of the illness, by emphasizing the physiological nature of the disorder. And, second, because depression is a complex illness in which the specific causes of the symptoms vary with each patient, my aim is to encourage health care professionals to examine and investigate the causes of depression in each case individually and to discourage existing preconceived notions about the nature of the illness.

CLINICAL DEPRESSION VERSUS THE BLUES

Recognizing that depression is a psychobiological illness is just one step in clarifying its nature. The dispelling of myths about depressive illness also necessitates the need to address the distinctions between normal and temporary depressed states from clinical depression.

Whether it is called dysphoria, a mood disorder, an affective disorder, dysthymia, unipolar disorder, depressive illness, or just plain depression, major depression can cause extreme distress that lasts for days, weeks, months, or even years. Just about everyone at some time in their life experiences fluctuations in mood and in emotions. People often become depressed momentarily, for example after failing an exam, or, conversely, feel a sense of elation and happiness after being offered a long sought-after job. However, there are some people who have mood disturbances and disorders and go through prolonged periods of extreme emotions, either depression or elation, sometimes both, which may not even be related to their present circumstances. Mood disturbances such as these can be upsetting and frightening because they can be disruptive to daily functioning and may even lead to suicidal behavior. This is clinical depression.

Because it is a term that is bandied about in everyday conversation, *depression* can generate some confusion; so, it is first important for all health care professionals to make a distinction between a temporary bout of feeling low or blue and the symptoms of full clinical depression. Depression can refer to a short-lived, negative feeling or a temporary mood state. This is the common understanding of depression. Brief bouts of feeling down are normal reactions to life's stresses and disappointments. This frame of mind or outlook can last a few hours or days or even weeks and it may seem intolerable and painful at the time. However, this mood eventually passes. Sometimes people reflect on and analyze their lives, their achievements, their prospects in very pessimistic, bleak terms. People at times have low opinions of themselves and decreased self-esteem. They lack confidence and motivation and fail to see that the future will bring any sense of happiness or fulfillment. As a result, they often become vapid and lack energy and begin to feel like they are living in a rut. But this phase also passes. They brave this turbulent period in their lives and sometimes can even learn valuable lessons about themselves.

However, as miserable as these experiences feel at the time, they do not penetrate to the very core of someone's existence. During such times, most people feel that they still have some sense of control over their lives and a more positive outlook and perspective is eventually regained. They know that they will get through these tough times. They will find a new job. They will fall in love again. Time heals those wounds.

Clinical depression, however, is very different and the variation in moods can be summarized in Figure 2. It is an illness comprising a specific set of symptoms that persist for certain periods of time. These symptoms are severe and cause quite a degree of distress. They will almost certainly disrupt the quality of life and impair the ability of affected individuals to function at work and in their relationships.

One of the main distinctions between brief episodes of unhappiness and clinical depression can be best thought of in terms

Severe depression

Moderate depression

Temproary low mood state | Normal
| Mood
Temporary elated mood state | Range

Bipolar II disorder

Bipolar I disorders

Figure 2.   Normal and abnormal mood ranges.

of being able to find comfort and relief from distress. When someone receives bad news, for example, it is normal to feel a sense of disappointment, loss, even anxiety. However, in these scenarios, even when someone feels devastated, he or she can often still find some support from friends or family or even in the realization that the situation, painful though it seems at the time, is temporary. However, if someone is suffering from clinical depression, no amount of sympathy, empathy, support, companionship, or encouraging words will provide comfort or solace. For most depressed people, the world is colorless, gray, and lacking in beauty. They of course can intellectualize that there are good things in the world, but they cannot *feel it*. They cannot appreciate it. The symptoms seem to be all-encompassing and what is particularly frightening and worrying is that all of their personality traits tend to be subsumed by depression. Before their illness, most people have unique personality traits, but depressed individuals tend to be remarkably and noticeably similar. They retreat into themselves. They become enclosed in a shell. Their suffering seems to be endless and the symptoms deplete them of every happiness or sense of well-being and security. As one of my clients, Christopher, recalls, depression disrupted his whole life:

> Even now, I can still remember struggling with the feelings of total hopelessness, despair, guilt. I had no energy, I was always tired. I couldn't eat, I couldn't sleep, I stopped seeing my friends. I felt like a total failure and just guilty, really, that I couldn't snap out of it. I was so frightened 'cause I didn't know what was happening to me. My wife even left me for a while. That's the thing about depression, it just attacks you on every level.

Dinah, another client, also reflects back on her own long battle with the illness:

> For me, I just remember most the feelings of being totally cut off from everyone else. It was like I couldn't connect with anyone else any more. It was as if a thick, smoky-gray glass wall separated me from everything and everyone else. There was no hope, only despair. Everything about my life looked bleak, miserable. My moods were all over the place, unsteady. Sometimes I would feel mentally okay, but physiologically depressed and so I thought I was becoming out of touch with my emotions. I also began to develop very extreme mood swings, as my emotional

state was always in constant turmoil. Mostly, as a result, all I wanted to do was to sink into a giant black hole and disappear altogether. Frankly, every night I hoped I would die in my sleep, so I would not have to wake up and face the painful consequences of yet another day. But, inevitably, every morning my eyes would open and I would feel the customary wave of anxiety at the thought of yet another twenty-four hours of misery and isolation from which I could not escape.

I also developed very severe panic attacks during this time. They were so terrifying. They would just hit me out of the blue and I would start to have problems breathing, my heart would pound, my palms would start to sweat, and I would generally become shaky, edgy, and irritable. By the time the panic attacks started to arrive with regular frequency, I was quite convinced I was cracking up. I was becoming emotionally unglued and it was absolutely frightening to feel so unstable; it was, without a doubt, a living hell. I felt any control over my life, my emotional equilibrium, my sanity were all just slipping away.

Providing a cohesive and more uniform understanding of clinical depression is problematic, not the least because the illness is shrouded in myths that complicate the process. Current definitions of the mood disorder tend to be laden with an emotional bias that is not only inaccurate, but also breeds stigma and fear. This goal of clarifying depression is further complicated because of a tendency for professionals and laypeople to assume that clinical depression is synonymous with the common everyday understanding of a temporary bout of the blues.

Since explanations about the nature of depression provide the foundation for investigations into the causes of the illness, biases, myths, and unsubstantiated claims about depression can mislead investigators and scientists into pursuing irrelevant research avenues, while other valid areas of research remain ignored. Chapter Four is the first of three chapters investigating the causes of depression and evaluates biological theories about the origins of the illness.

4

Biological Theories about the Causes of Depression

The last chapter dealt with some of the many problems regarding the origins of depression and demonstrated that myths about the illness abound and that there is a lack of consensus as to how the illness is defined. It should also be apparent that many scientists and health care professionals conceptualize depression as either biological or emotional and these conceptions then provide the framework for explaining the causes of depression. The myth that depression is *either* a psychological illness *or* a biological one then forms the basis to explain the origins of the illness. Since definitions provide the foundation for an inquiry, it is logical that the problems of definitions influence the ways in which people investigate the causes.

This stated, depression was not always viewed along these lines. Historically, the Egyptians and later the Greeks several thousand years ago themselves recognized depression and tried to explain its causes (see Gold, 1995). The Egyptians held the view that all illnesses, even emotional ones, had physiological causes and they believed that depression was the result of problems with the heart.

Hippocrates and other Greeks of the time argued that all ill health was the result of imbalances in the body's fluids or humors and depression was thought to be caused by an excess of black bile. But while our knowledge about the illness may have become more sophisticated and advanced through the centuries, neither the Egyptians nor the Greeks stigmatized patients with depression.

More recently, within the twentieth century, a tendency developed to separate the mind and the body especially for illnesses like depression, which is still evident today. Two men were largely responsible for this rigid distinction. Emil Kraepelin and Sigmund Freud were physicians who held the view that all mental health problems had a biological basis, although their treatment methods differed sharply. Freud's theories centered around the pathology of the human mind, and he believed that emotional problems could be resolved through talk therapy. Conversely, after many years of observing mentally ill patients on the wards of hospitals, Kraepelin emphasized physiological treatments. And, with these two eminent psychiatrists, the mind–body split begins.

GENERAL LIMITATIONS OF CURRENT THEORIES ABOUT THE CAUSES OF DEPRESSION

Clearly, explaining the causes of depression is a difficult task and there are many problems with the ways in which the disorder is conceptualized. Part of the problem rests with the tendency for scientists to rigidly view the illness as exclusively stemming from *either* biological *or* psychological causes. These lingering explanations, however, are outdated, mostly because they ignore the importance of the mind and body's dual role in the development of symptoms. But this tendency for some theorists to focus on psychological origins, while others concentrate solely on the biological can also lead to problems with diagnosis and treatment. And this is a potential minefield for anyone seeking help with depression. Many clients, because they think they have diagnosed the source of their depression, for example, a recent marital breakup, might immediately go to a therapist of some description and skip the visit to their physician. Therapists, themselves working from this rigid viewpoint, are not always adequately trained to point their client in the direction of a medical examination or insist that they first see a physician. In fact, most won't even recommend that their clients go to a physician at all.

There are many different theories about the causes of depression and they are rarely complementary; in fact, they are often in conflict with one another.

An obvious question is: Can any theory of the causes of depression account for all types and subtypes of the illness?

Scientists cannot answer this question with confidence at this stage in the research process, but many claim to do so. So, we must proceed with caution and there are some very important points that must be kept in mind when we are presented with any theory about the causes of depression. First, the theories that follow tend to focus on unipolar depression, but they rarely specify which subtype of unipolar depression they are explaining and explanations for the origins of other types of depression are largely ignored. Second, any credible theory of the origins of depression must also be able to explain the diverse symptom clusters that comprise physical, emotional, thought, and motivational characteristics. Moreover, explanations must also be able to account for the reasons for the onset of the illness and the maintenance of the depressive symptoms. Adequate theories must also offer us information on the episodic nature of clinical depression and offer valid accounts of why people will go into spontaneous remission and then redevelop the symptoms. Finally, these theories must also point to the reasons why some people, given similar circumstances and negative life events, fail to ever develop clinical depression. No doubt, this is a difficult task, particularly because there are probably many more subtypes of unipolar depression that have yet to be identified.

Because depression clearly and fundamentally affects the body's physiology, which is an area of research that is currently receiving the greatest attention, it is important to discuss some of the biochemistry of depression. This is also an area of research, broadly speaking, that is generating important information, discoveries, and breakthroughs, not only about depression, but also on how the brain and body work.

According to many researchers (for example, see Schuyler, 1974), there are several other important reasons why depression should be viewed primarily as a physiological disorder. Women often develop depressive symptoms before menstruation, after childbirth, and at menopause, which points to a hormonal problem, although again, we must be careful to avoid the stereotypes of depression as a woman's problem by turning normal biological functions into a pathological condition. Furthermore, when symptoms of depression are investigated across different cultures, there is some consistent evidence indicating biological causes, and somatic treatments—those that affect the body's physiology—such as drugs and electroconvulsive shock treatments are often effective in relieving symptoms of depression. It has also been found that symptoms can develop in nondepressed people as a result of the side effects of certain medications.

While depression clearly has a physiological basis, and much research is devoted to investigating the biological nature of the illness, it is essential that we address a number of limitations. First, research into physiological causes of depression fails to take account of psychological explanations about the origins of the illness. Second, the majority of studies focus on neurochemical imbalances. While no doubt brain structures are clearly implicated in many cases of depression, this almost exclusive attention to brain dysfunction means that other important physiological causes remain ignored.

NEUROCHEMICAL THEORIES
OF DEPRESSION

Depression is often described as being caused by a chemical imbalance in the brain, and much of the current research has found links between certain chemicals, called *neurotransmitters*, and mood disorders. Neurotransmitters, whose role is to send messages throughout the brain, are thought to be particularly important in causing depressive illness because one of their functions is to regulate mood. If levels of certain neurotransmitters become abnormally low, depression can occur; likewise, if these levels are too high, symptoms of mania can develop. Although several neurotransmitters have now been identified, many more have yet to be discovered, and research in this area is still very active. However, the discovery of the role of neurotransmitters in regulating mood and depression is important, because it has lent further credibility to the notion of different subtypes of unipolar depression and to the development of effective drug treatments.

The discovery of antidepressant drugs in the 1950s first provided the scientific community with essential clues about the role of neurotransmitters in regulating mood. Two particular drugs, called *tricyclics* (TCAs) and *monoamine oxidase inhibitors* (MAOIs), were found to be effective in relieving symptoms of depression. In what has been referred to as the catecholamine hypothesis of depression, the tricyclics, so-called because their molecular structure comprises three rings fused together, were found to block the absorption or reuptake of the neurotransmitter norepinephrine (noradrenaline). The second class of antidepressants, the MAOIs, prevent the enzyme monoamine oxidase from deactivating or breaking down the neurotransmitter. Both groups of antidepressants work by raising the amount of norepinephrine in the brain, leading to an elevation of mood.

Studying the brain is particularly problematic, because it is impossible to directly measure the levels of neurotransmitters, so that indirect methods are necessary and, unfortunately, somewhat crude. Researchers must resort to measuring substances known as *metabolites*, which are the by-products left behind after the chemicals break down. These metabolites can be found in body fluids, including urine, serum, and cerebrospinal fluid. For example, people who show low levels of the metabolite 3-methoxy-4-hydroxyphenylglycol (MHPG) have correspondingly low levels of norepinephrine. Conversely, for those with manic symptoms, we find high levels of this substance.

Although the discovery of the role of norepinephrine and neurotransmitters in regulating mood and causing depression was particularly groundbreaking at the time and continues to provide the framework for biochemical explanations of depression, the theory was soon found to have certain limitations. The prescription of tricyclics for people with low levels of norepinephrine was effective, but they did not work for everyone.

Later research led to several important discoveries. Other neurotransmitters were discovered and implicated in depressive illness, thus leading to the identity of more subtypes of unipolar depression. More recently, serotonin, another monoamine neurotransmitter that also regulates mood, was discovered. Because people with very low levels of this neurotransmitter exhibit more suicidal and homicidal tendencies, identifying serotonin was a major breakthrough. Scientists discovered that serotonin's metabolite, 5-hydroxyindoleacetic acid (5-HIAA), could be detected in cerebrospinal fluid and measured and eventually a new type of tricyclic drug, amitriptyline, was developed that selectively raised levels of serotonin instead of norepinephrine.

More evidence supporting the theory that these neurotransmitters were involved in causing depression came in the form of reserpine, a drug that is prescribed to treat high blood pressure. One of the side effects of reserpine, which was found to decrease levels of both norepinephrine and serotonin, was severe depression.

The discovery of both norepinephrine and serotonin and their role in regulating mood has been particularly important, not least because they provided solid evidence of the complexities of depression and that there are potentially very numerous subtypes of unipolar depression. The hunt is still on to discover and identify other neurotransmitters and more recently two in particular, acetylcholine and dopamine, are thought to have a role in depression.

Limitations of the Neurochemical Theory

While tricyclics and monoamine oxidase inhibitors and their impact on raising levels of neurotransmitters in the brain provide substantial evidence for the neurochemical hypothesis of depression, these theories are not without their limitations and more research is clearly necessary. The therapeutic properties of the drugs cannot result solely from increasing levels of neurotransmitters. On beginning drug therapy, there is an immediate increase in the levels of both serotonin and norepinephrine. However, after a week or so, the neurotransmitters are at their original levels, a finding not in keeping with the above hypothesis. Therefore, simply increasing levels of these neurotransmitters does not explain why these drugs help relieve the symptoms of depression.

But breakthroughs on research often lead to more unanswered questions. One discovery that has pointed to the limitations of the theory that increasing levels of both serotonin and norepinephrine alone will alleviate the symptoms of depression comes from investigations of more recent antidepressants. The drugs mianserin and zimelidine, for example, are seen to be effective antidepressants, but neither simply increases the levels of serotonin or norepinephrine.

THE NEUROENDOCRINE THEORY
OF DEPRESSION

As important as the discovery of the role of neurotransmitters in regulating mood is, at least at the present time, it can only serve as a partial explanation for what goes wrong physiologically when people become depressed. Thus, researchers began investigating other structures in the brain.

Other areas of research point to malfunctions in the neuroendocrine system of the brain that governs our hormones. This brain area implicates the limbic system, which governs emotions and includes the hypothalamus, which regulates the pituitary gland and the secretion of hormone levels. The pituitary is regarded as being particularly associated with the more "vegetative" symptoms of depression, including disturbances of appetite and sleep. Studies indicate that there is a strong relationship between the neuroendocrine system and depression, which should not be particularly surprising, because this is the body system that is most commonly associated with psychiatric problems, according to Gold (1995). In fact, problems with the neuroendocrine system are so important to the development of depression, it is now currently thought, that it has become an important diagnostic indicator.

The discovery linking hormones to depression was made fortuitously by Dr. Sachar, who was in the process of investigating the effects of psychotherapy in reducing stress levels in depressed patients. The focus of his investigation was the levels of the hormone cortisol, which is released in the bloodstream when we are under stress. He found that a majority of individuals with severe depression had increased levels of cortisol. When cortisol is released, a process of homeostasis is set into motion. Homeostasis refers to the mechanisms in the brain that maintain equilibrium and balance. For example, if we become anxious about something, the body immediately goes into a process of homeostasis, by dampening down the symptoms of anxiousness to restore the body to balance.

Endocrine glands are found throughout the human body; examples include the pituitary, hypothalamus, and pineal gland in the brain, the sex organs, the adrenals above the kidneys, and the thymus and thyroid gland located at the base of the neck. Endocrine glands produce hormones that regulate the body's chemistry and are secreted into the bloodstream. Blood pressure, body temperature, appetite, sexual activity and reproduction, growth and development, energy levels, heart rate, and response to stress are regulated by our hormones and they all work together to maintain the body's homeostasis.

Attached to the hypothalamus is the pituitary gland, which is thought to have a role in depressive illness. The posterior pituitary secretes two types of hormones, which are actually produced by the hypothalamus, but stored in the posterior pituitary. One is vasopressin, whose role is to activate the kidney to reabsorb water, and the other is oxytocin, which stimulates labor contractions. The anterior pituitary releases several hormones, including thyroid-secreting hormone (TSH), adrenocorticotropic hormone (ACTH), luteinizing hormone (LH), growth hormone (GH), prolactin (PRL), and follicle-stimulating hormone (FSH), which themselves are stimulated by hormones in the hypothalamus.

Because this gland is involved with so many hormones and has connections with the hypothalamus and the limbic system, when the pituitary malfunctions some people are likely to feel depressed.

Table 1 lists similarities between thyroid problems and depression. Researchers are now just beginning to understand the ways in which the neuroendocrine and nervous systems intertwine and write that they are undoubtedly influential in mood disorders for at least three reasons:

1. Certain neurotransmitters are also hormones. Norepinephrine and epinephrine are both adrenal hormones and neurotransmitters that are important mood regulators.
2. The same neurotransmitters regulate both the hypothalamus and mood.
3. Endocrine hormones, such as thyroid hormones, affect the neurotransmitters involved with regulating mood.

Table 1. Symptoms Shared by Hypothyroidism and Depression

Hypothyroidism	Common symptoms	Depression
Delayed reflexes	Depressed mood	Weight changes
Cardiac failure	Apathy	Appetite problems
Dry skin	Weight gain	Sleep problems
Brittle hair	Fatigue	
Loss of eyebrows	Impaired concentration	
Cold intolerance	Thoughts of suicide	
Goiter	Delusions	
	Decreased appetite	

SLEEP MECHANISMS AND DEPRESSION

The discoveries of neurotransmitters and the neuroendocrine systems and their role in regulating mood are important. Not only have they led to a greater understanding of brain functions in general, these discoveries also seem to unite and explain many of the physical and psychological symptoms of depression, a prerequisite of any valid, credible theory of the causes of mood disorders. However, although scientists are continuing to explore these areas, other research into human physiology is also generating important information about the nature of depression. One such area is that of sleep.

One of the cardinal symptoms of depression is a disturbance in sleep patterns, with people either sleeping too much or too little and experiencing disruptive sleep patterns throughout the night. Furthermore, people who are depressed receive fewer benefits from sleep, because their patterns are so shallow and fragmented. So, there does seem to be some obvious connection between sleep and mood disorders.

There are four stages of sleep in addition to what is referred to as rapid eye movement (REM) sleep, during which time we dream. Every stage of sleep and REM sleep is repeated at 90-minute cycles throughout the night. Normally, the deepest stage of sleep takes up the majority of the 90-minute time period at the beginning of the night and then becomes shorter as morning approaches. REM sleep, in contrast, takes up as little as 10 minutes per cycle early in the night but can become longer as we progress toward the time we wake up. But with depressed people, the pattern is reversed. REM sleep happens much more quickly after the individual first falls asleep and decreases toward morning. In fact, these sleeping patterns are so typical of biological depression that they are often used—or should be used—as a diagnostic aid. It has also been found that depressed people experience an increased number of rapid eye movements (Carlson, 1986).

Selective and Total Sleep Deprivation

In fairly recent years, a theory that has gained prominence is that one of the most effective "antidepressants" may be either selective or total sleep deprivation. Sleep deprivation of either sort, which is achieved by monitoring signs of REM sleep, seems to alleviate symptoms of depression. Similar to the effects of antidepressants, the therapeutic effect of selective sleep deprivation progresses slowly and develops and improves over the course of several weeks. Some patients continue to demonstrate long-term improvement even after they discontinue this deprivation.

Antidepressants also indicate that disturbances in sleep may contribute to or cause depression, for in addition to their pharmacological effects, these treatments suppress REM sleep, delay its onset, and decrease its duration. Somehow, then, REM sleep and mood dysfunction are connected.

Total sleep deprivation produces immediate antidepressant effects, unlike selective sleep deprivation, which takes several weeks to improve symptoms. So, when we sleep we produce a substance with a depressogenic effect, which can lead to depression. It is believed that this substance, which is produced in the brain, serves as a neuromodulator. When we wake up, we gradually metabolize this substance. Researchers found that some people who were deprived of sleep began the day depressed but then showed gradual improvements in mood throughout the day. This improved mood then continued through the next sleepless night and during the next day. However, when these individuals were finally permitted to sleep, their symptoms of depression quickly returned.

Why do some people who are depressed benefit from total sleep deprivation, while others do not?

This question cannot be fully answered yet, but Goodman, Wir-Justice, and Wehr (1982) discovered that one way to predict an individual's potential response rate is from his or her circadian pattern of moods. Circadian rhythms will be discussed in more detail below and refer to the regulation of our biological clocks. Just about everyone feels their best or better at one part of the day compared with another. Some people are morning people, while others seem to function better in the evening. People with depression also show these changes in mood. Research has found that people with depression who were most likely to experience the benefits of total sleep deprivation were those who complained of the worst symptoms in the morning and whose mood was better in the evening. They suggest that these people are most likely to feel the effects of the depressogenic substance that is assumed to be produced during sleep. This agent makes them feel particularly poorly in the morning, but as the day progresses, they begin to feel better as the chemical is metabolized. A sleepless night acts to further this improvement.

So, investigating sleep patterns seems to be a key to diagnosing depression among some people. But researchers still do not fully understand the reasons why we sleep at all. Although hypotheses have been put forth to explain the function of sleep, none has been conclusive. Some researchers claim that we inherited our need for sleep from our cavemen ancestors. It is argued that sleep ensured their survival by preventing them from stumbling around in the dark and injuring themselves or from being attacked and eaten by predators. Others argue instead that sleep has some restorative power that repairs our bodies and keeps our brain functioning, but these theories are just speculative at this stage. All we do know is that sleep is probably the strongest biological drive humans have. People can refuse to eat or drink, even for quite awhile, but most people cannot stave off the desire for sleep. Because disturbed sleeping patterns are cardinal symptoms of depression, and sleep is an important biological function, it is not surprising that scientists are investigating sleep dysfunction as a potential cause of mood disorders.

CIRCADIAN RHYTHMS AND DEPRESSION

That disruptive sleeping patterns are sometimes implicated in clinical depression may point to problems with some people's circadian rhythms. Our body is regulated by differing cycles and rhythms that are daily, monthly, lunar, and seasonal. Our need to sleep is governed by these cycles. The most basic cycle is the 24-hour day; the word *circadian* comes from Latin meaning about (*circa*) a day (*dies*).

In this way, rest and activity and sleep and wakefulness are all linked to body temperature and hormonal secretions and the smoothly ordered functioning of our biology is essential for both physical and mental well-being. So, during a 24-hour day, we experience a cycle of several physiological functions—heart rate, metabolic rate, breathing rate, body temperature—which all tend to be strongest during the late afternoon and early evening and at their weakest early in the morning. Monday morning blues and jet lag cause us discomfort, not because of loss of sleep, as it is commonly thought, but because our sleep cycles have been interrupted and need adjusting. A disruption of our daily clocks, even by a few hours, is enough to impair our concentration, energy, digestion, hunger, immunity, ability to repair tissue damage, stimulate healing processes, and mood (Gold, 1995).

How do circadian rhythms work? We still do not know for sure, but scientists currently believe that our biological cycles are determined by two oscillators working in harmony. One oscillator, which regulates and controls body temperature, secretions of some hormones, and REM or dream sleep, is thought to be strong and consistent. The other oscillator, which controls sleep and waking patterns, activity and rest, and sleep-dependent hormones, is thought to be weaker.

Both oscillators are tied to light and dark cues that are imposed from outside the body and these environmental signals ensure that they operate in tandem. If they are disrupted and become desynchronized for any reason, say through international travel, this can and does often create internal chaos because these cycles will have to readjust. Until they do, which can take a few days or even a few weeks, people are likely to feel out of sorts.

There does seem to be compelling evidence that depression for some people may be the result of a disruption in the circadian rhythms, which govern both oscillators, and that this episodic desynchronization of internal functions and environmental stimuli could account for many of the symptoms of depression. This is thought to be particularly true if hormonal secretions are out of sync.

Is there any evidence to support this viewpoint? Several experimental studies have been conducted with nondepressed subjects who were asked to spend some time in a room without windows or clocks to signal the time. In most cases, their day was seen to extend to 25 hours and they ended up with biological rhythms similar to depressed people. Furthermore, some even became depressed themselves.

Our internal clock is reset every day and it is thought that a tiny cluster of neurons, which are situated in the hypothalamus, tend to regulate these functions. Damage to a rat's suprachiasmatic nucleus (abbreviated SN or SCN) in the brain leads to a total disappearance of the circadian rhythm, and periods of eating, drinking, and sleeping, among others, become random during the 24-hour cycle.

The SCN is located directly above the optic chiasma, or the place where the two optic nerves connected to the brain meet. Nerve fibers are also connected to the hypothalamus and to the SCN, thus linking the external world with the brain's internal clock. More specifically, the light cues presented to the retina get passed on to the SCN, which regulates the sleep–wake cycle modulated by cues from the night and day. If this connection is impaired, the system becomes disrupted and dysfunctional.

The internal events that seem to lead us to crave sleep do rely to some extent on external cues. When nighttime arrives, the retina sends signals to the pineal gland ("the third eye"), whose role is to monitor the body's own cycles and to keep track of the external cues like light and dark. The pineal gland is responsible for secreting melatonin, which makes us feel sleepy. Another function of melatonin is to affect certain brain cells that make the neurotransmitter serotonin—also a sleep-related substance. Serotonin, in turn, is concentrated in the brain's raphe nuclei, which themselves produce a substance that induces light sleep. Therefore, serotonin may play various roles in its connection with depression.

In summary, several pathways seem to be joined here and scientists are continuing to research other brain structures to see how they are involved in the development of mood disorders. Gamma-aminobutyric acid (GABA), another neurotransmitter, has a role in anxiety, for example, and may be implicated in depression. Also, neuropeptides (sometimes referred to as *polypeptides*) are receiving some attention in the current literature. Neuropeptides help cells receive messages from the neurotransmitters and are themselves chemicals that share the properties of neurotransmitters and hormones. One example of a group of neuropeptides is the endorphins. Endorphins are sometimes referred to as the runner's high and have properties that reduce pain. Their role in mood and depression is currently being investigated.

To conclude, biological explanations for depression are far from simple or conclusive at this stage. In order to offer the most effective treatments possible to their patients and clients, health care professionals should continue to both keep abreast of the latest information on the complexities of brain structures and actively examine the newest discoveries.

5

Psychological Theories about the Causes of Depression

With so much research into the biological causes of depression, it might seem tempting to ignore the relevance of other theoretical perspectives. However, that would be shortsighted. The more traditional psychological theories, despite their many theoretical and methodological flaws, must also be considered. Because of the emotional bias so strongly associated with depression, psychological theories provide the basis for therapy and are profoundly influential in that regard. The aim of this chapter is to evaluate some of the more traditional and widespread theories as to the causes of depression. However, before introducing these therapies, I argue that it is more illuminating to group together some of the major theoretical limitations shared by these psychological explanations of depression.

There are many, often conflicting, psychological theories about depression. They tend to be outdated, anachronistic, and fail to incorporate breakthroughs and advances in the physiological understanding of depression. Furthermore, because they focus on the psychological aspect of depression, they ignore the psychobiological nature of the illness and instead focus exclusively on the emotional symptoms. Moreover, many of the psychological theories rely more on presumptions about human nature and depression than is borne out by scientific evidence. In addition, although these theories aim to explain the causes of depression, at best they address the symptoms of the illness. Finally, the major limitation is their sole emphasis on dysfunctional emotions as the cause of the illness. This emphasis on an individual's inability to cope with his or her personal catastrophes as the root cause of the disease, whether or not accurate or appropriate, can be misleading and interfere with treatment. As a result, these theories tend to place undue attention on a client's childhood and past relationships with his or her parents and mistakenly encourage neurotic tendencies and impulses. Although I would argue that some cases of depression are likely to have their origin in problematic childhoods and troubled parental relationships, there is clearly no evidence that the majority of depressed individuals belong in this category. Thus, for all of these reasons, psychological theories serve to confuse rather than clarify. And, in the process, they provide the foundations for stigma.

PSYCHOANALYTIC EXPLANATIONS OF DEPRESSION

As previously discussed, Freud was one of the psychiatrists influential in developing the idea of the mind–body split and although many psychological theories and approaches have been introduced since then, the emphasis on self-exploration of the past and childhood traumas remains particularly strong throughout psychology. Because of his widespread influence, Freud's attempts to find answers and order in the turbulent storm of the human mind have also influenced theories on depression.

Although there are many schools of psychoanalysis, Freud's remains the most renowned. The most traditional Freudian theoretical explanation conceptualizes depression as resulting from the real or imagined loss of a valued or loved object, through death, separation, rejection, or even symbolically through the loss of some ideal. In most cases, these "objects" represent individuals who are particularly important and significant, especially in early childhood. Mostly they signify a parent, usually the mother. Such a loss, according to this approach, predisposes the individual to later stresses if she or he is confronted with another major, significant loss, such as divorce or unemployment. In general terms, then, the emphasis of psychoanalytic theories is on the individual's long-term tendency to develop depression and not on the recent loss or stressors that trigger depression in many people.

The psychoanalytic view further suggests that because of the psyche's deeply entrenched belief that it is wrong to express anger at the loss or rejection of a parent, it instead turns the anger inward on itself. Such anger creates feelings of guilt and self-loathing.

In his famous work on the subject, *Mourning and Melancholia* (1917), Freud compared grief and depression, but he emphasized that in depression the important element is the loss of the individual's self-esteem. In his observations, Freud noted that depressed people exhibit certain symptoms that are like those seen when people mourn the loss of a loved one. However, unlike mourners, depressed people are more likely to be self-disparaging and lack confidence and self-esteem. It was his conclusion that the loathing is not directed at the self, but instead at the lost object or person.

He wrote:

> If one listens patiently to the many and varied self-accusations of the melancholic, one cannot in the end avoid the impression that often the most violent of these are hardly at all applicable to the patient himself, but that with insignificant modifications they do fit someone else, some person whom the patient loves, has loved or ought to love. . . . so we get the key to the clinical picture.

Other psychoanalysts have developed their own versions based on Freud's original theories and some should also be included here to illuminate the diversity of psychoanalytic approaches to conceptualizing the causes of depression. Moreover, most have similar themes. Klein (1935) claimed that an individual's tendency toward depression was the result of a problematic mother–child relationship in the first year of life and not the result of early childhood losses of a significant object. He argued that if the mother was unable to instill in her child feelings of being loved and secure during this time, the child would have greater difficulty relating to love objects and would thus be prone to depression. A tendency to develop depression, according to this view, is the result of an early inability to resolve depressive anxieties and to establish a healthy level of self-esteem.

Later variations of this "object relations" view come from Bowlby

(1973), whose research on early attachments in childhood has greatly influenced developmental psychology and in particular theories on infant social development. He stressed the importance of early bonding experiences between the infant and the mother as central for healthy psychological development. According to this view, disruptions in this process, by maternal deprivation or separation, could lead to problems for the individual later in life. Later research of course contradicts the rigidity of this claim. Attachments can be formed between the infant and a variety of caregivers including the father, siblings, grandparents, and family friends, and even disruptions of the attachment process resulting from separation do not necessarily lead to psychological ill health. Bowlby later reformulated some of his views.

Psychoanalytic views, although widely influential in conceptualizing depression, do have some limitations. For example, there is little experimental evidence to support their claims regarding the origins of depression. In addition, having been formulated several decades ago, psychoanalytic views are dated. Although some researchers (for example, Brown, 1979) have argued that the death of a mother during childhood will predispose her daughter to developing depression later in life, both depressed and nondepressed women are equally likely to have suffered the loss of a parent in childhood. The loss of a parent, particularly during childhood, is clearly a traumatic event, but other factors are necessary for the development of depression.

COGNITIVE THEORIES OF DEPRESSION

In recent years, the cognitive view of depression has become one of the most influential of the psychological theories of the illness. Cognitive theories emphasize thought processes as the most important cause of depression. In other words, the way in which the individual interprets and thinks about things is responsible for the development and maintenance of depression.

Generally speaking, the cognitive view emphasizes the ways in which depressed individuals think and how they view themselves and the world. Put simply, the cognitive perspective suggests that people with depression view themselves more negatively than do their nondepressed counterparts. Probably the most famous and influential of this type of theory of depression is that of Dr. Aaron Beck (1967). From his extensive clinical experience, Beck argues that people with depression exhibit certain irrational thought patterns in what he refers to as the *cognitive triad*: These individuals possess negative views of themselves, of their current position, and of their future possibilities.

The cognitive triad persists because depressed individuals tend to overgeneralize from their negative experiences. A common illustration of this is that depressed people tend to label themselves complete failures on the basis of a single disappointment. "I failed an exam, I must be completely stupid in everything I do." According to Beck, the existence of the cognitive triad is demonstrated by the ways in which depressed people misinterpret the events in their lives. Furthermore, depressed individuals tend to interpret an experience in a negative fashion, even when a more positive explanation is plausible. For example, if a depressed individual receives a promotion at work, he or she might attribute it to luck, rather than to good job performance. The depressed, according to these theorists, look for defeat and expect failure.

Origins of Faulty Thoughts

How do these faulty thoughts first arise? According to Dr. Beck, during childhood and adolescence, depressed people acquire *negative schemata* or thought processes through various events, including the loss of a parent, a personal tragedy, an illness, social rejection, or criticisms from teachers or parents. We all have schemata, many different schemata, which help us organize our lives, view the world. With depressed individuals, the negative schemata acquired earlier in life can become activated whenever the individual is exposed to new circumstances or situations that resemble, even tangentially, the conditions in which the negative schemata were originally learned. Furthermore, these negative schemata continue to be strengthened by and strengthen other biased thought processes, which lead to a distortion of reality. In this way, a negative schema that stresses incompetence can lead to expectations of failure and a negative self-appraisal schema emphasizes to the person that he or she is completely worthless. When these various negative schemata are combined with the cognitive biases, they maintain and strengthen the cognitive triad. The cognitive triad thus works in the following way:

1. *Arbitrary inference.* An individual reaches a particular conclusion even if the evidence to support it is limited or nonexistent. For example, such individuals might regard themselves as worthless because a traffic jam made them late for an important meeting—"Life is too much of a struggle. Nothing ever goes right."
2. *Selective abstraction.* An individual reaches a conclusion based only on one component of a particular situation. Having failed a test, the person considers himself or herself to be a dolt, despite the fact that half the class failed too.
3. *Overgeneralization.* An individual makes a sweeping conclusion based on a single, even trivial event. Not being hired, a job applicant is convinced that he or she is completely unfit—never acknowledging that several hundred other people had also applied for the job.
4. *Magnification and minimization.* This refers to an individual's tendency to exaggerate. In magnification, a scratch to a car might "destroy" the vehicle and make the individual "worthless." In minimization, an individual might believe that she or he is worthless despite successes at school and at work.

Beck's theory is unique. While many theorists see individuals as victims of their situations, Beck adopts the opposite position: that an individual's emotional reactions are connected to how he or she perceives the world. Depressed individuals are, in Beck's view, the product of their own illogical self-appraisals.

But despite enjoying tremendous influence in the understanding and treatment of depression, cognitive views of depression are not without their limitations. One of its main problems is the difficulty in determining whether the patterns of thought that typify depressed people are the cause of the depression or a result of the illness. Brewin (1985) offers some evidence that a negative thinking style accompanies the onset of depression. However, since negativity of thought is a classic *symptom* of the mood disorder, but not necessarily the *cause* of depression, cognitive therapies are not likely to be appropriate or effective for all clients.

BEHAVIORAL THEORIES OF DEPRESSION

In contrast to the cognitive theories of depression—which emphasize covert processes such as attitudes, self-assessments, images, memories, and beliefs—and to the psychoanalytic theories—which focus on early childhood loss and intrapsychic processes—behavioral theories instead stress that depression is caused through learning and environmental factors, and they focus on overt behavioral patterns and the social side of depression.

Developed in the 1950s and with many variations, the basic premise of this view is that depression is the result of a decrease in the degree of effective positive reinforcement sufferers receive from people in their social world, which lead to the onset and maintenance of depression. Although this decrease in the levels of positive reinforcement can be caused by many different things, most behavioral theorists stress either (1) problems with the individual's behavior which elicits negative feedback from others or (2) the low levels of reinforcement offered by others in the depressed individual's social world. Furthermore, the depression is compounded by the individual's sense of helplessness and inability to exercise or take control of his or her life subsequent to unpleasant experiences and traumas earlier in life. This sense of helplessness and lack of control is referred to as *learned helplessness.*

Despite the behavioral perspective of depression having been widely interpreted, many theorists fail to reach a consensus. In one version, developed more than four decades ago, B. F. Skinner regarded that depression was the result of weak behavior brought on by the disruption of typical patterns of behavior that had hitherto been positively reinforced by the individual's work and social environment. He referred to this as an *extinction schedule.*

Other theorists also agreed with this perspective of an extinction schedule as a cause of depression. Ferster (1975) wrote that depression resulted when a person no longer obtained the same degree of reinforcement from, for example, work or a partner. Depressed people are said to have problems adapting to this reduced reinforcement, which may itself be caused by numerous factors and changes in that environment. Since the individual must adapt and needs to acquire new sources of reinforcement, this may cause further difficulties. As a result, Ferster developed the theory of *chaining* that helps to better illustrate this process of generalization of the person's reaction to a more specific loss of reinforcement. The recent loss of a job, for example, could lead to reduced behaviors that were connected (or chained) to working. Thus, such a person might have problems waking in the morning, visiting friends or colleagues, planning and organizing daily activities, and so forth, if these behaviors and activities were organized around the job environment—which was the central core of this reinforcement.

Costello (1993), also behavioral theorist, suggested that a single source of reinforcement cannot easily explain the depressed individual's broader loss of interest in all things pleasurable. His view was, rather, that symptoms of depression were caused by a breakdown of the *chain behavior*, which is probably the result of the loss of one of the reinforcers in the chain. Furthermore, he held that the strength of the reinforcer depends on all parts of the behavior chain working well. When a chain of behavior breaks down in some way, there is a loss of the reinforcer effectiveness associated with all aspects of the chain. The reduction of reinforcer effectiveness, according to Costello, causes depression.

Lewisohn and others (for example, see Lewisohn *et al.*, 1978) devised their own behavioral theoretical perspective which is also influential in attempting to explain depression. Lewisohn's *reinforcement theory* is predicated on the belief that individuals with depression lack the necessary social skills to gain normal social reinforcement from others and as a result might even elicit negative behavior from others. For example, depressed people smile less and stimulate less smiling from others, receive fewer statements of support and more unpleasant facial expressions and more negative remarks from others than do nondepressed individuals.

Lewisohn *et al.* (1978) believed that depression is caused by a high rate of unpleasant or negative experiences and a low rate of positive reinforcement in the major areas of an individual's life.

They also argue that three main factors are particularly likely to contribute to these low levels of reinforcement. First, deficits in the person's behavior or skills prevent him or her from receiving positive reinforcers and/or lead to the individual's problems in coping with negative experiences. Widows or widowers and others who have experienced a similar form of social loss may have problems in forming new positive reinforcing relationships.

Second, a lack of potential reinforcers in the individual's environment may be the result of some social loss or an increase in negative experiences. The death or departure of people who provided social reinforcement or a recent unemployment may also lead to a lack of reinforcement. The third factor suggests that an individual becomes depressed if there is an increase in his or her sensitivity to negative events or a reduction in his or her ability to enjoy positive and pleasurable events.

Lewisohn and his colleagues stressed the importance of social skills to prevent depression in individuals. If an individual lacks social skills, he or she may have marked problems in attaining positive social reinforcement. Persons are seen as having good social skills if they can avoid negative consequences and elicit positive behavior from others in their social world. Because depressed people may lack positive reinforcement, they may also have difficulties in initiating and maintaining this behavior. As a result, they can become apathetic, passive, and withdrawn.

INTERPERSONAL THEORY OF DEPRESSION

A related theory, the interpersonal theory of depression, looks at the concept of social support and its connection with depression. Since many depressed individuals have limited socially supportive networks, they view themselves as having less support. This lack of social support seems to increase the person's inability to cope with stressful events. For example, in a study on homelessness (Downing-Orr, 1996) I discovered that homeless young people in London and in Sydney benefited tremendously from the social support of their peers on the streets and that the assistance, which came in the form of protection, food, money, friendship, acceptance, and accommodation, aided their survival.

An important question that needs to be addressed, though, is whether the lack of social support leads to depression or whether the depressed individual pushes away social support. Many depressed people have ineffective social skills, and some investigations have found difficulties solving interpersonal problems, problems maintaining eye contact, and problems with their speech. In addition, other investigations have reported that unipolar patients (Gotlib & Hammen, 1992) experience more stress and that their own actions add to these stress levels.

Furthermore, as others have argued, the depressed may elicit more negative reactions from others and they may have an offensive or awkward interpersonal style, which may elicit rejection from others.

However, as isolation and the desire to be alone are cardinal symptoms of depression, problems in relating well to other people are not necessarily the cause of the illness. Instead, a desire to be left alone, as a result of the illness, can lead to all kinds of social difficulties. In addition to social withdrawal, many depressed people are irritable, agitated, and short-tempered, or apathetic and uninterested in making an effort to accommodate others, which in turn causes relationships to break down.

THE COGNITIVE–BEHAVIORAL PERSPECTIVE

Some theories of depression combine cognitive and behavioral explanations. One example of this is an updated version of the learned helplessness theory, called the *learned hopelessness theory*. It seeks to explain why some people who are depressed feel they have no control over their lives. Seligman (1989b) holds that this belief results from experiences in which the individual has little control or power over the thoughts or events in his or her life. While the perception that one has little or no control over life does not automatically lead to depression, Seligman suggests that depression comes about as a result of the way people interpret these events in their lives. Depressed individuals are more likely to explain negative experiences using stable, global, and internal factors (Abramson *et al.*, 1978). A stable factor is something that is unchangeable, a global factor refers to something that influences almost all aspects of an individual's life, and an internal factor focuses not on the environment but on the individual.

Some investigations have found that depressed individuals are predisposed to viewing negative events in their lives by the above three factors. For example, using learned helplessness theory to look at student scholastic achievement, a depressed student would most likely explain a poor grade on an exam using internal, stable, and global factors. Thus, the poor performance means he or she is unintelligent and will continue to receive poor grades on all future tests.

The most recent update of this theory is the learned hopelessness theory. Abramson *et al.* (1989) suggest that some types of depression are the result of an individual's state of hopelessness. According to this view, these people expect that desirable outcomes will not happen to them and/or that undesirable ones will inevitably occur. Furthermore, the depressed feel unable to exercise influence over the events in their lives and, as a result, develop a profound sense of hopelessness that leads to depression.

While negative life events often lead to distress and can trigger clinical depression, it is also important to remember that a profound sense of hopelessness about oneself, the future, and one's ability to take control of one's life are all *symptoms* of depression and do not necessarily signal the *cause* of the illness. So, while it may be tempting for a health care professional to view a client's feelings of inadequacy and hopelessness in the wake of a personal catastrophe as the sure cause of the depressed symptoms, an acceptance of them at face value, without any further investigation, could lead to ineffective and inappropriate treatments and continued suffering.

STRESS AS A CAUSE OF DEPRESSION

Stress as a health problem has received an enormous amount of attention in recent years and has been implicated as a cause of depression. Stress is now accepted as a harmful side effect of modern life. According to Dr. Hans Selye, an expert in the field, stress can be defined as the body's physiological response to psychological and physical demands. The detrimental effects of stress on physical and emotional well-being have been researched and documented. When people feel the negative side of stress, they are not coping well with their lives and high stress levels are likely then to have harmful consequences. Some of the many ways in which stress takes its toll on health are depression, asthma, ulcers, diabetes, dizziness, nausea, indigestion, racing pulse, trembling, rheumatoid arthritis, hypertension, and, most seriously of all, heart disease, stroke, and even cancer.

Because studies on stress have indicated a whole host of related health problems, researchers have also made the link between stress and depression. Since it is commonly held among health care professionals that depression can be caused by a personal catastrophe or negative life event, such as a recent bereavement, a job loss, or the breakdown of a close relationship, and because these stressors can be debilitating, it is reasonable to assume that they can trigger clinical depression. But do they?

According to one study, death rates among the first-degree relatives of recently deceased men and women in Wales were significantly higher than average, presumably reflecting the heightened combination of stress and mourning (Milligan & Clare, 1994). Furthermore, Paykel (1979) argued, based on the results of another study, that depressed patients reported experiencing a particularly stressful event in their lives a few months before the onset of their symptoms (Paykel, 1979), although the specific events that were more likely to trigger depression were not identified. However, the same author argues that some stressful, yet positive life events—such as winning the lottery, getting married, even going on holiday—can lead to depression, so perhaps it is the stress induced by an event, rather than the specific event, that triggers the depressive episode.

Furthermore, some investigations have found that depressed people have histories of more trauma during childhood and of more loss, and frequently more life stressors within a year or two of the actual onset of depression. A British academic, Brown (1979), conducted a very famous study of women in London. He found that women were much more likely to report depression if their mother had died before they were 11 years old and also if recently they experienced a loss that was particularly severe. Death of the mother after the age of 11 or death of the father at any time does not seem to be a risk factor.

While the emphasis on negative life events as triggers for depression has a certain amount of commonsensical, intuitive appeal and there is much evidence that stressful situations alter the body's chemistry, there are also some limitations to the view that stress causes mood disorders. First, vast numbers of people who experience childhood difficulties and later losses and stressful events do not go on to develop clinical depression. Furthermore, many depressed people report having had *no* early childhood or recent stressful events. So, while personal setbacks can be upsetting, most people eventually get over them without developing clinical depression.

In the light of conflicting evidence, the role of stress as a causal factor of depression is in need of clarification. Perhaps we need to study why some people become depressed in the face of trauma while others do not. In my view, some people are likely more vulnerable to a depressive response following a stressful event because of certain vulnerability factors or in the face of some provoking agent or even because of long-term chronic problems. All of these can trigger depression, because the physiological changes produced by stress can lead to abnormally low levels of neurotransmitters. This disruption of normal functioning is then further impaired by the individual's perception of reduced control over his or her situation. So, while stress can alter and impair our physiology and contribute to depression, individuals' perceptions about their empowerment and their ability to make improvements is also an important ingredient.

In summary, this chapter has examined some of the more influential psychological theories on the causes of depression. Several limitations of the theories have been discussed. Because they largely assume that emotional causes are to blame, these theories serve to perpetuate the myth and imply that depressed people are personally inadequate to cope with life's pressures. Furthermore, they ignore the biological origins of depression and fail to explain the fact that depression could be a normal reaction to life's circumstances, have a productive value, or be symptomatic of another health problem. Such is the focus of Chapter Six.

6

Alternative Theories about the Causes of Depression

Although the more traditional and accepted physiological and psychological theories about the causes of depression have been influential and illuminating, it should also be evident that there are several theoretical and methodological limitations to many of these explanations. The most glaring limitation of these theories is that they are rigidly based on the assumption that depression is *either* a psychological illness *or* a biological one, so that other potential areas of explanation are ignored. Neurochemical malfunctions, childhood traumas, or poor social skills fail to explain Shelly's intolerance to a combination of caffeine and sugar. Furthermore, there is evidence to suggest that in some circumstances, depression is even an accurate, realistic response and reaction to a troubled life. Therefore, in order to offer better theoretical accounts of depression, it is essential to accept that physiological causes of depression are not limited to the neurochemical and that existential crises and despair are also relevant. Although there are no doubt numerous and thought-provoking alternative theories about the origins of depression, two in particular are discussed below.

ALTERNATIVE THEORY NO. 1: DEPRESSION IS AN ACCURATE RESPONSE TO A TROUBLED LIFE

One of the main limitations of psychological therapy is its insistence that human distress is a sign of breakdown or pathology. In the Introduction, I argued that the social psychological concept of the Fundamental Attribution Error was relevant and, at least in part, responsible for the tendency of many health care professionals to hold patients and clients responsible for their problems, which creates stigma. Nowhere in clinical psychology is this bias more glaring than in depression.

This stated, however, according to existential philosophy, misery, disappointment, angst, and despair are part and parcel of the human condition and, as such, philosophers do not apportion blame to the troubled individual. It is my view that health care professionals can learn a great deal about mood disorders and the depressed person from the teachings of existential philosophy. Some people have more tragic and traumatic circumstances in their lives than others and in many situations pessimistic and negative views of the world are both relevant and an accurate reflection of their personal catastrophes. Perhaps then, instead, some people could be challenged for having an overly optimistic view of life?

One researcher held this belief. Lauren Alloy (1988) concluded that nondepressed people tend to look at the world through rose-colored glasses because they have a tendency to overestimate the likelihood that positive events will happen to them and ignore the likelihood of negative events. Perhaps, then, nondepressed individuals possess an overly unrealistic positive view of themselves and the world, whereas depressed people, in contrast, are more objective and painfully accurate in their view of their life.

ALTERNATIVE THEORY NO. 2: DEPRESSION CAN BE A PRODUCTIVE RESPONSE

An alternative theory of depression comes from Emmy Gut (1988). She argues that depression can actually be beneficial by serving as a productive response to a negative life situation:

> Whenever we perceive, largely unconsciously, that a significant physical or psychological effort of ours is failing in its purpose or coming to a halt, and we cannot grasp what is amiss, we react with an (emotional) response that I call "the basic depressed response". Like all (emotional) responses, it is accompanied by a set of typical psychological symptoms.

According to this view, depressive symptoms are seen as the normal result when people face some inner conflict or inner deadlock that seems unresolvable and they may remain depressed until the problem is overcome. Gut argues that a temporary bout of depression which most people experience from time to time is different from major depression. While the basic depressed response is similar in both cases, that is, it is a result of the inner conflict, the temporary depressive succeeds in locating internal and external resources to resolve the problem, whereas the depressed individual is unable to resolve the problem. Furthermore, depressive-proneness in an individual is the result of unfavorable patterns in childhood produced by problematic interpersonal relationships and cultural pressures. "When being depressed does not facilitate a process leading to a successful outcome, one needs to identify what impedes this intrapsychic task and to assist the patient in overcoming the obstacles."

In order for Gut and other similar-minded therapists to determine whether an individual is suffering from a healthy or a pathological depressed mood state, she evaluates the "adaptive" or "maladaptive" effects of her client's crisis in relation to the individual's personal, psychological, and environmental triggers of the crisis. Basically, she looks at the person's life and the events leading up to the crisis. She writes of "productive depression," which refers to the end of a depressive episode, during which something useful or beneficial has been learned by the individual, some personal development or growth has been achieved, behavioral patterns reorganized, and, following the depressed period, the individual functions more effectively in attaining some goal or even becomes more realistic in defining goals and objectives. "Unproductive depression," according to Gut, refers to those circumstances in which learning and adaptation have been promoted, but no personal growth or development has been achieved and health deteriorates.

While it is perhaps difficult to conceive of depression as ever being productive or normal, particularly when people are suffering from the misery of the symptoms, this perspective can be useful and insightful, because it means that people can actually learn something valuable and positive from their depression and their illness can lead to personal growth and development. Being depressed forces many people to take stock of their lives and to rediscover what it is that they may want to achieve. Gut writes on the process of this self-discovery:

> When after having been depressed we find ourselves relieved from feeling incomprehensibly slow and ineffective, we often feel new vigor, have some new ideas or plans or we suddenly understand what has been wrong, we may find that we actually have more cause than we earlier recognized for anger, grief, regret, humiliation, disappointment or other discomfort. Or we may see that in an important issue we may have been barking up the wrong tree. Such insights are accompanied by feelings appropriate to whatever was the cause for the hidden discomfort. Since our depressed mood and symptoms have vanished at that point, we may not see them as connected in any way with our new ideas and plans, our recovered vigor, or with new insight into our situation.

But, instead, many tend to think of depression as weak and undesirable. Perhaps practitioners should try to help their clients view their episode or episodes of depression as a similar emotional response to grief, anxiety, or anger when they are in their appropriate context.

So, as Gut argues, depression has been traditionally thought of as an emotional or mental illness caused by heredity, as a faulty personality trait that prevents the individual from coping with intrapsychic or psychological conflict, as a lack of the ability to cope with social stress, or as the result of biochemical disturbances in the brain. Whatever the initial causes of the illness, for many people mood disorders can signal a positive and beneficial change. Depression, according to this theory, can lead to a better intuitive grasp of a personal situation or difficulty and lead to resolutions, growth, and maturation.

ALTERNATIVE PHYSIOLOGICAL CAUSES OF DEPRESSION

While theories about depression that view the illness as either an accurate reflection of someone's personal circumstances or a productive way to cope with an intrapsychic deadlock are just two of the ways in which it is possible to broaden the theoretical debate on the causes of depression, there are other explanations that are equally valid. Previously, Shelly's case history demonstrated the interaction between sugar and caffeine intolerance and symptoms of depression and anxiety. Once isolated and identified, Shelly's symptoms were easily cured, despite their severity and disabling effects.

As a practitioner, I have helped many clients overcome and cure themselves of depression and, based on my experience and expertise, I argue that emotional symptoms often are not automatically indicative of mood disorders. In fact, according to a study conducted by the U.S. Department of Health and Human Services, as much as a third of psychiatric patients are being treated for emotional illnesses that they do not have, because the true physiological cause of their symptoms remains undetected (Gold, 1995). In the following pages, I discuss some of the more common neurological, physiological, and pharmacological imitators of depression. This discussion should, therefore, provide ample evidence that health care professionals must broaden their understanding of the causes of depression. The imitation occurs in at least five important ways, which demonstrates why it is not always easy to distinguish between mood disorders (or primary depression) and other illnesses (or secondary depression) that present with emotional symptoms:

1. Physical illness can magnify emotional problems. Researchers report that the more serious or chronic a physical illness, the greater the emotional distress to which it leads. One of the main reasons why individuals continue to suffer a relapse of emotional symptoms or fail to respond to psychiatric intervention is that the physical illness remains undiagnosed.
2. A patient with a previously existing physical illness can develop emotional problems as a result. However, this type of depression is usually temporary and disappears when the patient recovers.
3. A patient can have both psychiatric and physical illnesses that are unrelated to one another. Treatment of the physical illness then will have no beneficial effect on the psychiatric.
4. Emotional illnesses may cause physical illnesses. Because

depression is seen to weaken the immune system, the individual's ability to fight physical diseases might be compromised.

5. Some emotional disorders are the result of physical illness. Thus, treating the physical illness will lead to recovery from the emotional symptoms.

As the evidence suggests, people who have emotional symptoms may actually be suffering from an underlying physical disorder and not from a mood disorder. Since some of the cardinal symptoms of depression such as weight loss, fatigue, appetite disturbances, and problems with sleep are also indicative of other diseases, a physical illness other than depression must first be ruled out. These are often regarded to be mimickers of depression. According to a study conducted in a London general practice, almost 25% of patients with severe symptoms of depression were found to have a concurrent physical illness that was believed to be at least a partial cause of the depression (Milligan & Clare, 1994).

Earlier, evidence was put forth to show that symptoms of neuroendocrine disorders, such as hypothyroidism, may at times be confused with those of depression. Other illnesses such as some types of cancer often first appear in a patient as depression. In addition, certain drugs for illnesses like high blood pressure, allergies, and epilepsy can trigger depression. Since it is often assumed by health care professionals and the patients themselves that long-term disability or chronic illness profoundly affects the quality of life and therefore depression is a by-product, they come to accept these symptoms as inevitable.

There are several known mimickers of depression. In an earlier chapter, the neuroendocrine theory of depression illustrated problems caused by thyroidism and demonstrated that depressive illness and thyroid disorders have many common symptoms. Unfortunately, many of the diseases can be serious and if doctors and health care professionals address depression when the actual cause of the emotional symptoms is some other life-threatening health problem, valuable treatment time is lost. Furthermore, in some cases, otherwise innocuous mimickers cause emotional symptoms, which can be quite distressing and severe. While the causes might not be life threatening, the emotional impact can be disturbing and even increase a person's risk of suicide. The unpleasant emotional symptoms and risk of suicide can be eliminated by investigating and identifying the cause, thereby curing the emotional distress.

Tables 2 through 11 summarize some of the many physiological causes of depression that are not commonly investigated by health care professionals.

DISEASES OF THE CENTRAL NERVOUS SYSTEM

While Tables 2 to 11 summarize some of the many physiological causes of depression, it will be illuminating to discuss some of these factors in more detail. I begin with the role of the central nervous system in causing depression. Since evidence of emotional distress in patients is often automatically diagnosed as clinical depression, the actual cause of symptoms can remain undetected and, therefore, untreated. There are several illnesses or even injuries to the central

Table 2.   Neurological Causes
of Depression

Demetias (including Alzheimer's)
Epilepsy*
Fahr's syndrome*
Huntington's disease*
Hydrocephalus
Infections (including AIDS and neurosyphilis)*
Migraines*
Multiple sclerosis*
Narcolepsy
Neoplasms*
Parkinson's disease
Progressive supranuclear palsy
Sleep apnea
Strokes*
Trauma*
Wilson's disease*

*Produces manic symptoms as well.

Table 3. Endocrine Causes
of Depression

Adrenal (Cushing's,* Addison's diseases)
Hyperthyroid
Hypothyroid
Menses-related*
Parathyroid disorders
Postpartum*

---

*Produces manic symptoms as well.

nervous system, for example, that are often mistaken for depression. Because many of these diseases affect elderly patients, many health care professionals assume that depression is the real problem, reflecting their biases that older adults are more likely to be depressed because of generally deteriorating health, imminent death, loss of independence and status, and other bereavements. Unfortunately, a delay in diagnosing problems of the central nervous system can prolong suffering, lead to further deterioration, and impair the effectiveness of later treatments.

Dementia

Dementia is one such problem related to the central nervous system. Since the deterioration is pathological, this illness affects the brain and impairs its function, often permanently. Although dementia mostly afflicts the elderly, it can sometimes be evident among

Table 4. Infectious and Inflammatory
Causes of Depression

AIDS	Sjogren's arteritis
Bacterial pneumonia	Temporal arteritis
Lupus*	Tuberculosis
Mononucleosis/glandular fever	Viral pneumonia
Rheumatoid arthritis	

---

*Produces manic symptoms as well.

Table 5.   Miscellaneous Medical
Causes of Depression

Cancer (especially pancreatic and stomach)
Cardiopulmonary disease
Kidney diseases
Porphyria
Vitamin deficiencies (B_{12}, C, folate, niacin, thiamine)*

*Produces manic symptoms as well.

younger people, usually as a result of drug abuse, alcoholism, diabetes, or kidney failure.

Because emotional distress can be a symptom of dementia, this illness is often first misdiagnosed as clinical depression. To compound the problem further, it is estimated that as many as 50% of elderly patients with dementia may also be suffering from depression.

In some cases, the elderly patient is misdiagnosed as having depression, when in fact he or she has dementia. Because of this mistaken diagnosis, the elderly patient receives treatment for a non-existent illness and is denied therapy for the symptoms of dementia. Although there is no cure for this illness, the patient can still receive benefits from a proper diagnosis and treatment.

Table 6.   Analgesic and Anti-Inflammatory
Drugs as Causes of Depression

Analgesics/anti-inflammatories	Antibacterials/antifungals
Ibuprofen	Ampicillin
Indomethacin	Cycloserine
Opiates	Ethionamide
Phenacetin	Metronidazole
	Nalidixic acid
	Nitrofurantoin
	Streptomycin
	Sulfamethoxazole
	Sulfonamides
	Tetracycline

Table 7.　Antihypertensives/Cardiac Drugs
as Causes of Depression

Alphamethyldopa	Guanethidine	Procainamide
Beta blockers	Hydralazine	Quanabenzacetate
Bethanidine	Lidocaine	Rescinnamine
Clonidine	Methoserpidine	Reserpine
Digitalis	Prazosin	Veratrum

Alzheimer's Disease

Alzheimer's disease, which afflicts millions of elderly people, is a form of dementia. As for dementia, Alzheimer's disease is often first misdiagnosed as clinical depression, because a large number of Alzheimer's patients also present with emotional symptoms.

While there is no cure for Alzheimer's, a proper diagnosis early in the course of the disease means that patients can receive some available treatments such as drugs to improve memory and to reduce agitation.

Head Injury or Trauma

Head injuries and traumas related to postconcussion syndrome can also produce emotional symptoms, which lead to a misdiagnosis of depression. Injuries or traumas to the head, particularly to the frontal lobe region, can lead to severe changes in personality, including depression, anxiety, mood swings, and outbursts of rage. While these symptoms are often associated with major head injuries, even a mild blow can produce symptoms of anxiety, fatigue, irritability, and depression sometimes several months after the accident. In their

Table 8.　Antineoplastic Drugs
as Causes of Depression

Azathioprine (AZT)	Trimethoprim
6-Azauridine	Vincristine
Bleomycin	

Table 9. Neurological and
Psychiatric Drugs as Causes
of Depression

Amantadine	Neuroleptics
Baclofen	Phenytoin
Bromocriptine	Sedatives/hypnotics
Carbamazepine	Tetrabenazine
Levodopa	

initial assessment or preliminary examination, therefore, health care professionals should determine whether the client/patient has received any blows to the head prior to the onset of the depressed symptoms.

Multiple Sclerosis

Multiple sclerosis is another central nervous system disease that is often first misdiagnosed as depression. Multiple sclerosis, which usually strikes men and women between the ages of 20 and 40, refers to a chronic and deteriorating condition in which the sheaths surrounding the nerves break down.

In addition to the physical and neurological symptoms that typify this illness, psychiatric symptoms are also likely to develop. These psychiatric symptoms include emotional outbursts and distress, euphoria, and depression, and because they are temporary and intermittent, they are often mistaken for depression. A misdiagnosis of depression can have serious ramifications for future treatments and can impair the quality of the patient's health. Although there is

Table 10. Steroids and
Hormones as Causes
of Depressions

Corticosteroids	Prednisone
Danazol	Triamcinolone
Oral contraceptives	

Table 11.   Miscellaneous Drugs
as Causes of Depression

Acetazolamide
Choline
Cimetidine
Cyproheptadine
Diphenoxylate
Disulfiram
Methysergide
Stimulants (amphetamines, fenfluramine)

no cure for multiple sclerosis, new medications can delay its progress and deterioration and should be prescribed to maintain muscle
strength.

Parkinson's Disease

Parkinson's disease, which tends to afflict the elderly, is another
such illness. It is a progressive and debilitating disorder, with physical and psychiatric symptoms, for which there is no cure.

Physical symptoms include an involuntary tremor in the hands,
which gets worse when the patient is agitated or anxious. Facial ex-
pression often becomes flat, with unblinking, staring eyes. Posture
becomes stooped and patients often acquire a shuffling gait. Walking
also becomes difficult and many patients have great difficulty getting
started, but once they have begun to walk they find it difficult to stop.

Before the onset of the physical symptoms of Parkinson's, many
patients first develop emotional ones, which can lead to a misdiagnosis and a delay of treatment.

LEGAL AND ILLEGAL DRUGS

Drugs, whether legal or illegal, prescription or over-the-counter,
are widely available and used. Although they are usually taken for
their beneficial properties, there may be unpleasant side effects. The
drugs influence and change the body's chemistry and some side

Table 12. Recreational Drugs

Drug	Depressed symptoms	Manic symptoms
Methadone	✓	
Heroin	✓	
Sedatives	✓	
Cocaine	✓	✓
Amphetamines	✓	✓
Marijuana	✓	✓
PCP	✓	✓

effects can include emotional distress. Table 12 lists some of the more widespread types of recreational drugs that produce symptoms of depression.

Because drugs interact with and can impair the brain's mood regulating systems, they can dramatically alter the way we feel. Although the pleasant effects of the drug are temporary, the brain's chemistry can be altered for much longer periods. If an individual abuses the substance regularly, it can actually substitute for the natural chemicals in the brain. The brain may respond by ceasing to produce the chemicals or, compared with the powerful effect of the artificial substances, the brain's natural chemicals may seem weaker. Depression is often evident in substance abusers, along with anxiety and even psychosis. Sometimes the effects are irreversible, permanent brain damage having resulted.

Prescription Drugs

Psychiatric symptoms are not just the preserve of illegal substances and can occur with use of prescription drugs. In the early 1970s, researchers found that about 3% of people developed psychiatric symptoms from the drugs they were prescribed; today, because so many more medications have been introduced into use, the percentage is undoubtedly higher. Such symptoms include, in addition to depression, anxiety, emotional distress, hallucinations, psychosis, excessive tiredness, nervousness, nightmares, and delusions.

The prescription drugs that can lead to depression include certain cardiovascular drugs, hormones, psychotropics, anticancer agents, anti-inflammatory agents, barbiturates, anticonvulsants, and corticosteroids. Even antidepressants can cause depression if they are removed very suddenly.

Nonprescription Drugs

Many over-the-counter drugs can produce psychiatric symptoms of depression and occur more frequently than people imagine. Diet pills, cold and cough suppressants, and laxatives can have this effect. The culprit chemicals tend to be phenylpropanolamine, ephedrine, pseudoephedrine, and aminophylline.

Alcohol

Because of its widespread acceptance and its use as a social lubricant, many people forget that alcohol use and abuse also have depressogenic effects. According to Gold (1995), although there is evidence that alcohol consumption has declined in the United States since the mid-1980s, estimates are that over 100 million people consume alcohol. It is the prevailing belief that many individuals abuse alcohol because they are depressed and need an outlet for escape. However, it many cases, the depressed symptoms are in fact caused by alcohol consumption.

In terms of treatment, many alcohol abusers are first treated for their depression, usually in the form of antidepressant drugs. However, researchers have found (Gold, 1995) that when the alcohol problem is seen as the primary problem and focus for treatment, the symptoms of depression disappear once the effects of the alcohol leave the person's system.

NUTRITIONAL PROBLEMS

Shelly's case (Chapter Two) illuminated the role that dietary factors can have in triggering symptoms of depression. Certain food substances, in particular caffeine, sugar, and spices, act as stimulants that can cause mood swings.

In addition, nutritional deficiencies and toxicity can also mimic depression to which certain groups of people, especially the elderly, are more prone. Deficiency of the B vitamins, which help in brain metabolism in particular, can produce depressive symptoms, and this deficiency is quite common. For example, a study of a British hospital psychiatric unit found that over 50% of admissions had vitamin B deficiencies. Although treating this problem is quite straightforward and easy, the failure to do so could result in permanent neurological or psychiatric damage. The B vitamins include niacin, folic acid, B_{12}, B_6, B_2, and B_1. Vitamin C deficiencies can also lead to symptoms of depression.

Essential Metals/Minerals

More commonly called *minerals*, essential metals include sodium, potassium, magnesium, calcium, vanadium, chromium, manganese, iron, cobalt, copper, zinc, molybdenum, nickel, strontium, and selenium. Minerals are important to the body's physiology because they aid in enzyme functioning and metabolic processes. Insufficient levels of these minerals, reflecting malnutrition or metabolic problems, could produce a deficiency. Conversely, if an individual's intake of minerals is excessive, toxicity or poisoning can occur. Psychiatric and emotional symptoms, either from toxicity or from deficiency, are numerous.

Low Cholesterol Intake

Studies have long indicated that a no-fat diet may be beneficial to health by reducing overall risks of heart disease, although a low cholesterol intake may also cause symptoms of depression and increase the risk of suicide. A study of over 300 people who attempted suicide but survived found levels of cholesterol in their blood to be significantly below those of a comparable nonsuicidal group.

Physicians have questioned why dietary programs designed to reduce heart attack deaths have failed to decrease the incidence of overall deaths. According to some studies, the decrease in heart attacks has been met by an increase in deaths from accidents, murder, and suicide.

In 1995, the *British Medical Journal* reported that Italian re-searchers found a link between low cholesterol levels and depression and aggression. The evidence indicates that low cholesterol levels affect the brain's capacity to absorb serotonin, one of the important neurotransmitters affecting mood and regulating harmful impulses.

CANCER

Major depression is a common symptom for many different types of cancer. It is estimated that up to 50% of cancer patients also develop depression. Because cancer is a life-threatening illness, it is essential to rule out this disease when a patient appears to be de-pressed. People who fail to respond to psychiatric medication and who have lost a great deal of weight in particular may be suffering from cancer and not depression. Common cancers can include lung, pancreatic, carcinoid syndrome, and central nervous system tumors.

INFECTIOUS DISEASES

Several infectious diseases often produce symptoms of depres-sion. These include mononucleosis or glandular fever, which is caused by the Epstein–Barr virus. Epstein–Barr is a herpesvirus that attacks the white blood cells whose role it is to combat illness. The symptoms can be manifold, ranging from mild to severe, including a sore throat, swollen glands, headache, fatigue, and general weak-ness. Because the virus can spread to many organs in the body, diagnosis may be difficult and the risks of complication are in-creased. In about 50% of patients, the spleen becomes enlarged, increasing the risk of rupture. Depression may develop and it may be one of the most lingering symptoms.

Chronic Fatigue Syndrome

In recent years, chronic fatigue syndrome ("yuppie flu") has attracted public interest. The illness has also been linked to depression and shares many of the same symptoms, leading to confusion and misdiagnoses.

The main symptom of chronic fatigue syndrome is excessive tiredness, which can last for months or even years. Other symptoms include headaches, fever, and concentration problems, and a number of patients are unable to maintain a job or even carry out simple functions of life, such as shopping. Because the illness has been found among people in isolated areas, it has led researchers to conjecture a viral cause.

Mood symptoms that are associated with chronic fatigue syndrome can be confused with depression, but antidepressant treatments for chronic fatigue syndrome have not been promising although they have reduced some symptoms.

ENVIRONMENTAL POISONS

The toxicity of chemicals, waste, and pollution—consequences of our modern age and its contamination of the environment—can harm people and cause depression.

Carbon Monoxide

Carbon monoxide is a highly toxic gas, which is both colorless and odorless. Because the gas is present in cigarette smoke, car exhaust fumes, and when we burn wood, charcoal, or coal, most people are exposed to carbon monoxide on a regular basis. However, its poisonous effects are felt only after a long exposure.

Carbon monoxide affects the body by depleting it of oxygen and, when poisoned, people respond in many different ways. Exposure to carbon monoxide has produced symptoms of depression, psychosis, schizophrenia, and hysteria, among others.

Organophosphate Insecticides

Organophosphate insecticides interfere with the essential brain enzyme acetylcholinesterase, and their effect on the human body is similar to that of nerve gas. Prolonged exposure to organophos-phates can lead to a whole host of distressing symptoms including anxiety, irritability, fatigue, giddiness, concentration problems and confusion, restlessness, and depression. The Countess of Mar was recently reported (*London Evening Standard*, May 3, 1996) as suffering from long-term depression after getting sheep-dip inside her boot. Because of her extreme symptoms, she has launched a campaign to ban these insecticides.

Solvents

Solvents in paint, gasoline, cleaning fluid, and glue can trigger symptoms of depression. Although most of the damaging effects of these solvents disappear when exposure to them is removed, other symptoms include fatigue, personality changes, hallucinations, irri-tability, and panic.

The aim of this chapter has been to demonstrate the need for researchers and health care professionals to broaden their under-standing of the causes of depression. Although biological causes are clearly relevant, most physiological theories focus on neurochemical dysfunctions and ignore the many other physiological, pharmaco-logical, and neurological triggers of depressive symptoms. The lim-itations of the psychological theories are too numerous to repeat here, but they tend to equate depression with a personal inability to deal with life's difficulties and disappointments. Because of the in-herent bias explained by the Fundamental Attribution Error, health care professionals fail to acknowledge that depression can, in certain circumstances, be a realistic reaction to life's catastrophes.

In isolation, these theories would merely provide the founda-tions for debate among academics and other scientists. However, in terms of patient care, the definitions and explanations as to the nature and origins of depression—limitations and all—provide the basis for diagnosis and treatment.

II

Current Problems in Diagnosing Depression

7

Diagnosis
A Problem of Stereotyping

Section One pointed out some of the many glaring inconsistencies in the way depression is currently defined and explained and it should be of little surprise that these theoretical flaws also influence the ways in which mood disorders are diagnosed.

Although depression is a complex illness or represents a wide variety of different health complaints, emotional symptoms receive the most focus, leading to the bias that depressed people are morally weak, emotionally unstable, and unable to cope with life's disappointments. This bias in turn leads to stigma.

Whereas there is ample research into the biological causes of depressive illness, as most of the investigators are researchers rather than practitioners, there is usually quite a long delay before patients receive the benefit. Conversely, the majority of psychological theories, because they have been developed and refined by therapists, tend to have a more immediate influence on treatment. As a result of this bias, several problems are introduced in the diagnosis of depression. In the first instance, since depression is viewed not so much as an illness but a moral statement about someone's character, the disorder tends to be diagnosed on the basis of stereotypes, as certain people are seen as more prone to depression than others.

In addition, depression tends to be diagnosed on the basis of patient self-reports and explanations for their symptoms. Because most physicians and nonmedical professionals dismiss the need to administer objective laboratory tests to confirm or rule out conclusively depressive illness, the diagnostic process tends to be subjective. However, as discussed in the last chapter, since emotional symptoms can be indicative of other serious health complaints, these subjective diagnostic methods tend to be rife with mistakes. With most other major illnesses, whether cancer, heart disease, diabetes, or AIDS, physicians and other health care professionals seek objective evidence confirming the cause of symptoms before prescribing treatment. With depression, however, the symptoms are accepted at face value.

RISK FACTORS OR STEREOTYPING?

If it is possible to conclude anything about depression, particularly in terms of risk factors, it is that depression can afflict just about anyone. No one is immune from its debilitating effects, and, as discussed in the Introduction, the disorder is quite common. According to the National Institute of Mental Health, those at highest risk are people between the ages of 25 and 45, although children and the elderly are also prone to the illness.

This stated, the evidence suggests that some people are more likely to develop depressive illness than others. One way physicians and other health care professionals diagnose depression is through risk factors or increased vulnerability to developing the illness. However, while the evidence does suggest that some people have a greater tendency to develop the disorder, mental health professionals could be relying too much on stereotypes of certain people to make their diagnosis. Since most clinicians are middle-class, middle-aged, white males, there is every likelihood that certain types of people, who differ from the clinicians, can be labeled as depressive and this can also seriously affect their diagnosis and treatment.

Genetics and Depression

Much of the current research is now focusing on the relationship between genetics and depression, and the tendency for people to inherit the disorder receives much support in the literature. Since physiology is known to have considerable impact on mood and mood disorders and physical problems are part of the symptoms of the illness, it is a logical progression for scientists to look for biological origins of depression and mania. In fact, research is pointing to a genetic link in both depression and anxiety. An investigation conducted both in the United States and in the United Kingdom has found evidence that genetic characteristics can determine anxiety and thus that some individuals are biologically more susceptible to developing symptoms of anxiety, but these investigations are still in their embryonic stages.

This discovery, should it be conclusively confirmed, would have important ramifications for those suffering from depression. Evidence that depression was in some way inherited would be further proof that this illness has a physiological basis and would serve to reduce the stigma that is so often associated with the illness. Furthermore, since the symptoms of depression are so multifaceted, a genetic predisposition would help explain their diversity and also give us important clues as to why some people, when faced with similar opposition in their lives, do not develop clinical depression.

Is there any other evidence that depression is inherited?

The most obvious way to determine if a predisposition to develop depression is inherited is through family studies and it is in these investigations that researchers try to determine the relative importance of a person's biology compared with the environment. There does seem to be a link between families and depression. If a family member has a unipolar or bipolar disorder, the risk is seen in some studies to increase among first-degree relatives to two to three times higher than normal. Some studies have also found that if one parent and a sibling suffer from depression, there is a 25% increase in the chances that another child in the family will also suffer from depression. This rate increases to 40% if both parents and a sibling have depressive symptoms.

The Amish Study

In order to study the link between depression and genetics, researchers have conducted some interesting studies of heritability estimates or the relative influence of both genetics and the environment. Janice Egeland and her colleagues (1987) examined chromosome structures of family members of patients diagnosed with bipolar disorder. By studying the Amish, who are an ideal group for such investigations because they tend to marry within the same community, she discovered a common genetic defect on the tip of the short arm of the eleventh chromosome. However, because only about two-thirds of those who inherit the gene actually go on to develop the disorder, environmental factors are also influential. Follow-up investigations of other relatives of bipolar patients, however, have not yielded the same results and have not confirmed these findings. Thus, Egeland's results may signal that there are different subtypes of bipolar disorder, some of which are connected to this chromosome.

Twin Studies

Researchers have also turned to twin studies for evidence of the relative influence of the person's environment and genetics. If one identical twin develops depression, there is a greater likelihood that the other one will too. And, because they come from the same egg, this seems to provide evidence of genetics. But, we cannot say so for certain. Some studies estimate that identical (monozygotic) twins have a 40% concordance rate, compared with 11% for fraternal (dizygotic) twins, thus pointing to the importance of genetics.

If the tendency to develop depression were entirely genetic, however, the concordance rate would be 100%, so biology and genes do not alone trigger depression. Professor Robin Priest, who is chairman of the Defeat Depression campaign in Britain, has argued that genetic factors only account for 50% of an individual's vulnerability to developing depression.

In terms of diagnosis, physicians and other health care professionals might be tempted to diagnose depression when they take a patient's family history. However, while many studies point to a genetic basis for depression, scientists need to address the relative influence between genetics and environment in developing depression and to question the role genes and biology play with mood disorders. The tendency for family members to develop depression may, in fact, reflect not so much their genetic heritage, but more the household in which they were raised.

Gender and Depression

While genetic influence seems to play some role in depression, a biological cause of mood disorders seems to be the acceptable face of depressive illness. However, other vulnerability and heightened risk factors can lead to stereotyping and stigma. Women, the elderly, and certain ethnic minorities, in particular, seem to fall prey to this method of diagnosis.

In terms of gender and depression, there is an almost universal observation that women are much more likely to exhibit symptoms of unipolar depression than men. Academic research has revealed that women seem to be more vulnerable to unipolar depression than men and almost twice as many females are treated for the illness than males. It is commonly held that varying life stresses, childbirth, learned helplessness of women, and hormonal effects are to blame.

But are these conclusions or are they stereotypes of female behavior?

Some other data also seem to support this claim. A similar two-to-one female-to-male ratio was found in door-to-door surveys of men and women in British urban areas and this same two-to-one ratio seems to hold in other cultures, in Europe as well as in the United States and is also evident in two villages in Uganda (Orley, 1970).

In another investigation, large numbers of men and women were compared as to income, employment, age, marital status, head of household, and so forth. It was found that in all but two categories, more women than men reported symptoms of depression.

Why are women more likely to suffer from depression?

Several attempts have been made to explain why women tend to suffer more from depression than men. In the first instance, women are probably more likely to express emotional distress than men in our and other societies, according to many theorists. When women experience loss, for example, it is culturally more acceptable for them to cry, while men are more likely to respond with anger or indifference, reactions that are not considered typical for depression.

Other proposed explanations for women's biological vulnerability to depression include chemical enzyme activity, genetic predisposition, childbirth, hormonal disturbances, and the monthly menstrual cycle.

Other academics claim that this tendency is related to the theory of helplessness, as discussed earlier. This theory suggests that because women learn to be more helpless than men, depression will occur more often in females.

In her investigations of factors that influence the persistence of depressive episodes, Nolen-Hoeksema (1987) claimed that the differences in gender may be attributed to the different ways men and women cope with depression. Men typically respond to depression by engaging in activities that will distract them from thinking about their mood, for example, watching television, playing a sport. By contrast, women are seen to be less active (a bias with out justification in my view) and more likely to mull over their situation and blame themselves for being depressed. This rumination is seen to increase the depressed state and negative mood, perhaps by preventing women from attempting to solve their problems.

Many other studies support this theory. Individuals who revealed that they tend to mull over problems are less likely to try to solve their problems (Nolen-Hoeksema, 1987). Furthermore, this tendency to ruminate on their problems, instead of actively trying to find solutions for them, is associated with longer bouts of depression. This reflects how people cope with depression rather than the reasons for their depression.

A feasible question to ask is whether women tend to adopt this mulling tendency in response to sadness and stress compared with their male counterparts. Nolen-Hoeksema suggests that the answers could lie in childhood and the way men and women learn sex roles. She suggests that masculinity is associated with coping and being active and not engaging in an analysis of one's problems and feelings. In contrast, little girls learn that they are more emotional by nature. Because depression has emotional symptoms, by definition, it is more natural for girls and women and is unavoidable.

The feminist perspective would argue that the greater tendency for women to become depressed is the result of their lack of personal and political power. Their perspective claims that more women become depressed because their social roles do not encourage them to feel competent. A woman's contribution to society does not seem to be valued compared with the greater power men have.

In my view, all of these factors might be relevant for some women, and indeed, many can apply to certain men. However, many of the existing theories do point to the overreliance on stereotypes of women. Women are helpless. Women are emotional. Women cannot handle their hormones. Women are weak. Women cannot cope. Women are powerless in society. Women's work is undervalued. However, there are three salient criticisms with this view that women are more likely to develop depression than men.

First, if health care professionals assume women are more likely to suffer depression, then they will find evidence to support their prejudice. Since they are not looking for symptoms of depression in men, physicians and psychologists fail to diagnose the problem in that population.

Second, the entire assumption that women who seek help for their emotional problems are weak and demonstrating their inability to cope is itself a prejudice without merit. People who monitor and assess their physical and emotional well-being and seek treatment when problems develop are, in fact, exhibiting responsibility and concern about their health.

Third, the evidence now suggests that men and women are equally likely to suffer from depression. However, women are more likely to seek treatment than men; and, while women complain of emotional symptoms, men are more likely to report physical symptoms. For example, in a 5-year study of teachers, Wilhelm and Parker (1989) found no gender differences in depressive episodes. Since there were no role differences in terms of occupation between male and female teachers, gender proneness to depression may be connected to social factors.

How do men cope with their symptoms of depression?

Unfortunately, depressed men tend to be more self-destructive and this is also dangerous to their health. According to a recent study, because men are reluctant to show they need help, they are more likely to try to escape from their worries through drunken and aggressive behavior, abusing drugs, or even working extended hours. The British Royal College of Psychiatrists, who conducted this study, even suggests that underdiagnosis of depression in men may be as high as 65% and that when men do go to their physician it is likely to be with the more physical complaints of depression, which the physician will accept at face value.

The importance of these findings, though, cannot be over-emphasized because a person's diagnosis and treatment are likely to depend on how he or she is perceived by the physician. If a woman is perceived as a greater candidate to develop depression, because she is emotional and has difficulty coping with life's stressors, she might be automatically referred to a therapist without further investigation of her symptoms. Likewise, perhaps symptoms of depression in men, if they are more likely to complain of the physical ones, remain undetected because men are seen as emotionally stronger and more resilient. It would appear, then, that stereotyping of both sexes is relevant and leads to problems in diagnosis.

Age and Depression

According to many studies, depression among adults seems to increase with age in terms of both severity and frequency. It is argued that depression is particularly prevalent among middle-aged women because of endocrine changes related to menopause, the empty nest syndrome, children growing up and leaving the house, fears of growing old, and doubts about sexual attractiveness. In addition, there is a sense of helplessness associated with the elderly and de-pendence induced by physical and mental incapacity.

Again, descriptions such as these sound more like stereotypes, particularly of elderly women. Old people are confused. Old people are lonely. Old people are close to death. So, of course, they are more depressed. But, are they? According to research, the elderly are not any more likely to become depressed than younger people, (Gold, 1995), and they are less likely than young adults to suffer from mood disorders (Eaton, Kramer, Dryman, & Shapiro, 1989). In fact, many elderly patients with depression are likely to have a long history of the illness.

Certain illnesses associated with the elderly, however, may also share symptoms of depression. For example, depression could be symptomatic of Alzheimer's or dementia. Furthermore, elderly patients with strokes to the left hemisphere of the brain may also suffer feelings of despair. While we still do not have a full understanding of how the brain works, some investigators have claimed that positive emotions, like happiness, are associated with greater activation in the left hemisphere (Davidson *et al.*, 1992) and that negative emotions are centered in the right hemisphere. Support for this theory has been found in studies of brain-damaged patients (Levanthal, 1980): Those with injuries, including strokes to the left part of the brain, the happiness center, revealed more symptoms of negative emotions, including crying and pessimism.

While the common belief is that depression increases with age, several studies are instead suggesting that rates of depression among younger people are growing. According to Dr. Paul Harris of Oxford University, although it was once believed that children did not become depressed, newer evidence has shown that symptoms of depression in children are very real.

It has been estimated that up to 6 million children may be afflicted with depression, which has been undiagnosed and thus untreated, again pointing to the danger of relying on stereotypes of age.

Race, Social Class, and Depression

There are no firm conclusions that people from certain ethnic or social backgrounds are any more likely to suffer from depression. However, while the prevalence of depression is not seen to have a racial vulnerability, there is a tendency for physicians to overdiagnose symptoms of schizophrenia and underdiagnose mood disorders in patients from different racial and cultural backgrounds and again this points to stereotyping by clinicians.

Social and economic class position was also not likely to be a factor in vulnerability to depression, because everyone, despite social position or material wealth, can be prone to developing symptoms of the illness. According to some studies, those who are financially disadvantaged may show more feelings of hopelessness and powerlessness, while their more economically empowered counterparts may show a greater likelihood to feel rejected and lonely, pessimistic and socially isolated. So, they are equally likely to be depressed, but perhaps for different reasons.

Are Some People More Prone to Developing Depression?

In my view, many factors are likely to play an important role in determining whether someone is vulnerable to developing depression; and this is what health care professionals must understand instead of relying on stereotypes of certain individuals. Someone's genetic heritage and biological makeup, other mental or physical conditions, nutrition, stress, childhood experiences and traumas, relationship difficulties, career problems, timing, and the lack of coping resources may interact and trigger depression. For some people, biology alone might be enough to trigger depression; for others, the inability to contend with a painful experience; but for many others, it is likely to be a combination of things. Depression is such a complex and multifaceted illness and an acknowledgment of these many different factors will more likely lead to a better diagnosis and treatment strategy.

While the process of diagnosis becomes problematic because of an overreliance on stereotypes of individuals, further complications in this procedure occur because of a tendency for health care professionals to diagnose on the subjective basis of their patients' self-reports of their symptoms.

8

The Subjectivity
of Symptoms

Health care professionals begin to form a diagnostic picture of a patient or client based on stereotypes of individuals whom they believe will be more likely to develop depression. However, the diagnostic process further breaks down when the patient describes his or her symptoms. Although patients should be encouraged to describe their symptoms and offer an explanation about the likely cause of their health disturbances, relying exclusively on the patient interview and his or her self-reports renders the diagnosis subjective.

The aim of this chapter is to challenge the tendency of health care professionals to focus exclusively on the emotional nature of the illness by presenting and discussing the other cardinal symptoms of depression and to demonstrate the reasons why diagnosing depression on the basis of symptoms alone is inadequate.

DIAGNOSING SYMPTOMS
OF DEPRESSION

Although it is tempting to equate emotional distress exclusively with mood disorders, because depression is a psychobiological illness, its symptoms also affect the person's physiology, motivation, and concentration. Certain very specific criteria are recommended for diagnosing the illness. Making sense of clinical depression can be complicated, because it comprises a whole variety of symptoms, which can vary greatly, sometimes with no specific feelings of melancholy at all—not all depressed clients feel sad—to different types of symptoms with varying degrees of severity.

The symptoms listed in Table 13 reveal the wide range of very diverse symptoms that plague people with depression, although most people tend to equate one symptom—feelings of extreme sadness—with the illness. So, health care professionals must look out for a wide range of symptoms in addition to mood.

For the majority of people, though, the main problem associated with depression is a disturbance of mood where they feel down and are unable to enjoy the pleasures they had previously experienced. For many, their thought patterns change, become distorted, which affects how they view themselves, the world, and the future. Depressed people often have terrible self-esteem problems, feel guilty

Table 13.   Symptoms of Depression

Mood or emotional symptoms	Thought symptoms
Feelings of misery	Negative self-appraisal
Lack of self-esteem	Hallucinations
A sense of hopelessness	Bleak outlook for future
Unhappiness	A sense of failure
Shame	Thoughts of inferiority
Worthlessness	Inadequacy
Downheartedness	Useless
Humiliation	Incompetent
Uselessness	Thought distortions
Guilt	Suicidal thoughts
Extreme sadness	Self-blame
Excessive crying	Concentration difficulties
Feeling emotionally flat	Thought disturbances
Loss of pleasure	Death
Inability to enjoy anything	Memory problems
Irritability	Self-loathing
Motivational symptoms	Physical symptoms
Apathy	Appetite disturbances
Lack of motivation	Sleep disturbances
Inertia	Fatigue
Boredom	Anxiety and panic
Discouragement	Bodily aches and pains
Lack of control	

and worthy only of punishment. Lack of motivation, or apathy, might be construed as evidence of this failure. Most believe they are no longer likable, lovable, attractive, or good company and see themselves as somehow personally defective and think they will always be this way. Depression alters intellectual functioning and affects one's memory and ability to concentrate and make decisions.

Depressed people tend to develop negative self-assessments about their abilities and their worth and as a result tend to avoid the company of others. And so the vicious cycle continues and the person becomes more negative. Negative self-appraisals then become the norm and self-esteem becomes increasingly more deflated. Many people erroneously think of themselves as inferior, failures, inadequate, useless, and incompetent. More profoundly, they also tend to believe that they are the source of their failures, but these perceptions are normally just distortions of thought.

Furthermore, depressed people often feel tremendous guilt and blame themselves for all of their problems. When they fail at something, such as getting a job, they tend to think the worst—that they will never get a job. Even when they do achieve some sort of success, they often dismiss it as some sort of fluke, and believe that in no time at all they will be found out to be the failures they are convinced they are. In extreme cases, people believe they are responsible for all of the world's problems.

The future is usually only viewed in terms of great pessimism. In fact, the depressed individual has a stockpile of responses to justify the belief that the future will hold nothing but pain. But distortions of thoughts are also very common with depression. Personal qualities and strengths seem impoverished and insignificant and even happy memories of past events become transformed into the negative and the unpleasant.

Depressed people often feel irritable. Perhaps they turn to friends who cannot offer the support or sympathy the individual wants and requires; and because a depressed person often feels unworthy and hopeless, this contact may only serve to reinforce his or her unlovable qualities.

In some cases, depressed people report a profound inability to feel pleasure or enjoy anything about life and this loss of pleasure may exist with or without symptoms of feeling down or melancholy. Hobbies, recreation, and other interests all seem to lose their appeal. It is as if everything becomes flat and dull.

Apathy and lack of motivation are also problems associated with depression. Depressed people lose their motivation, sometimes even their will to live. Most people face their day. They wake up and have breakfast, go to work or to school, seek entertainment and the company of family and friends. People with depression have great difficulty getting up in the morning.

People with depression often turn to thoughts of suicide and death and suicidal and parasuicidal behavior among the depressed is quite common. Estimates show that 1 in 20 depressed people will take their own life (Gold, 1995). Depressed individuals think of death constantly and have a preoccupation with ending their misery. They may believe that the only way to gain relief from their illness is through suicide or they think that their family and friends will be better off if they are dead.

Physical symptoms also accompany depression and as the illness progresses they can become worse. Changes in appetite are common. In some cases, people lose their appetite altogether, and may have to force themselves to eat, in order to avoid malnutrition. In other cases, people experience an increased desire to eat. Sometimes eating patterns alternate; patients have no appetite at all, particularly during anxious times or panic attacks, but then on other occasions, they crave certain foods, especially sugar, which can further contribute to their mood swings.

Some depressed people also report bodily symptoms, which may or may not accompany symptoms of melancholy. Backaches, headaches, dizziness, general malaise, gastrointestinal problems, even bleeding gums, and countless others also signal a mood disorder.

Many report psychomotor changes, including agitation or an inability to sit still, evidence of pacing, hand-wringing, rubbing or pulling of skin, or psychomotor retardation, including slowness of speech, in thinking processes, body movements, pauses in speech, and a decrease in the inflection and tone of the voice.

A lack of energy and increased tiredness are also present. An individual may feel tired even if there has been no physical exertion.

For these people, even the smallest task requires much energy and effort. Efficiency may be greatly reduced. For example, getting dressed in the morning may take a lot longer than normal.

Sleep disturbances are also typical. Some people develop insomnia, others fall asleep initially but experience early morning wake-ups and cannot fall back asleep. Others need sleep more. These physical signs are particularly profound. Not eating or sleeping properly can magnify other symptoms of depression and lead to malnutrition, irritability, and thought, concentration, and memory problems. Libido also diminishes. Further studies even report that depressed individuals may be more susceptible to illness, because depression may have detrimental effects on the immune system.

With respect to friends and family of the depressed person, they will often continue to view him or her as they did before the depression arose. If depressed individuals do complain about being unhappy or express fears of being unsuccessful, their grumblings are likely to be dismissed as irrational, perhaps even overdramatic. Those with depression might be regarded as attractive, intelligent, and sociable but that does not mean they hold that view of themselves. Sometimes even when families and friends witness these changes in personality and self-perception, they do not think they are permanent—just going through a bad time, a rut, they reason. Those closest may also feel confused and fail to comprehend the full profound extent of what the depressed person is feeling and why his or her outlook is so bleak. Shelly was often told that she was being overdramatic, negative, unreasonable and her fears and worries were dismissed, by even the people closest to her.

The Problems with Relying on Symptoms as a Method of Diagnosis

There are many different problems associated with a diagnosis based on patients' self-reports about their symptoms. First, although there are many physical, motivational, and concentration disturbances, physicians and other health care professionals tend to focus almost exclusively on the emotional symptoms. Because some people do not feel tremendous and profound sadness when they are depressed, or, particularly in the case of men, emphasize the physical nature of their symptoms, there is the danger that many health care professionals are failing to diagnose the illness. Furthermore, because many of the symptoms of depression are similar to those of other illnesses, relying exclusively on symptoms as a method of diagnosis means that patients can be treated for an illness they do not have. For example, hallucinations can be a symptom of severe depression, but can also indicate drug abuse or schizophrenia. Finally, perception and description of symptoms vary widely among the depressed. If such individuals are feeling particularly apathetic, they may have little energy or interest in detailing how they feel, while others may be particularly agitated and irritable. Furthermore, some depressed people, particularly those who have been suffering for a prolonged period, may have become accustomed to their symptoms so that they actually seem normal. In short, there is very little consensus even among depressed patients about their symptoms.

In order to overcome problems with these ambiguities, many health care professionals use the *Diagnostic and Statistical Manual* (DSM-IV) as a guide in interviewing patients about their symptoms. Although the manual's questions can help the diagnostic process by serving to prompt and to remind patients of their symptoms, it is by no means problem free. Typical questions are reproduced in Table 14.

If the depressed individual answers yes to at least five of these questions and if these symptoms have persisted most days for at least 2 weeks, then some form of depression is likely. The most important feature of a major depressive episode, at least in terms of diagnosis, however, is the time frame. An individual must have had the symptoms on most or all days of at least a 2-week period before depression is diagnosed. DSM-IV is the bible of the psychiatric and psychological professions and many individuals are diagnosed based on answers to questions such as these. And, on close inspection of these questions, they do seem to cover quite adequately many of the main symptom clusters that typify depression.

However, the DSM method of diagnosing depression is not without its critics, and these criticisms are important for anyone who is treating people for clinical depression. The DSM system of diagnosis can lead practitioners down the wrong pathway, because of its

Table 14. Diagnosing Symptoms of Depression

1. Do you feel a profound sense of sadness, hopelessness, or despair?
2. Have you lost interest in the activities that normally give you pleasure?
3. Have you noticed a significant change in your appetite, either eating less or more?
4. Have you developed problems or changes in sleeping patterns, either sleeping too little or too much?
5. Do you feel lethargic and apathetic?
6. Do you feel excessively tired and drained of energy?
7. Are you experiencing a persistent sense of hopelessness or guilt?
8. Are you suffering from problems in your ability to think or concentrate?
9. Are you contemplating suicide?

Adapted from American Psychiatric Assoication (1994).

emphasis on behavioral symptoms. The DSM points to the dysfunction of the mind, when a physiological or medical cause may be more relevant, as we saw with Shelly. And this is an important point for all health care professionals. There is a long-established tradition in medicine to divide symptoms into two main camps: either emotional spheres, for the psychiatrist or psychologist to deal with, or physical ones, for the internist. As a result, physicians and psychologists often fail to rule out any organic, physical dysfunction as the cause of depression.

Furthermore, while the DSM description of symptoms may indicate that a person is suffering from depression, the symptoms can equally be the first ones of a serious health problem or even be reactions to a prescription drug, an illegal substance, or a mineral deficiency. There are at least 75 diseases and probably more that first manifest themselves through emotional symptoms.

There are three other problems with the DSM system of diagnosis:

1. The criteria are too broad and descriptive and can be applicable to more than one disorder.
2. This can cause problems because the treatment and the diagnosis may not be appropriate or accurate.
3. The DSM fails to include the cause of the disorder.

In summary, the DSM method of diagnosing depression, in many cases, leads to a tendency to overemphasize the psychological and emotional problems with depression and minimize other potential factors and causes. So, while the DSM aims to simplify and facilitate the diagnostic process, it instead often leads to an inaccurate diagnosis.

9

Problems in Classifying Depression

The final step in the diagnostic process tends to involve determining if the patient is suffering from major depression, dysthymia, or bipolar disorder. This phase is also subjective and rife with limitations. The potential for inaccuracy and misdiagnosis is related mainly to the persistent myth that depression is either a problem of emotions or of the anatomy and the failure to acknowledge the interlink between the body and the mind.

Since most practitioners explain the origins of depression as either a biological or a psychological disturbance, they also rigidly classify the illness in very much the same way. Once they have determined both that symptoms are present and for a period of at least 2 weeks, most clinicians then continue the diagnostic process by determining whether physical or emotional causes are to blame and so rarely look for possible alternatives. However, although this diagnostic process is logical, even commonsensical, because most practitioners tend to emphasize the *wrong* category classification, they can unwittingly jeopardize their patient/client. Instead of first determining whether the person suffers from primary or secondary depression, health care professionals tend to determine causality by looking at external or internal factors and at the unipolar or bipolar categories. And this is the second mistake most practitioners make.

In most books on clinical depression, it is categorically stated that depression is caused by *either* internal *or* external factors and that depression is *either* a unipolar *or* a bipolar illness. However, these categories should only be viewed as heuristics or guidelines for diagnosis, because there is no conclusive evidence that they even exist. Furthermore, because most health care professionals fail to distinguish between primary depression, which is the illness, and secondary depression, in which symptoms indicate another health problem, overrelying on these two categories is often misleading in terms of both effective diagnosis and treatment. While they have an intuitive, commonsensical appeal about them, there is little conclusive scientific evidence, if any, that depression can be reliably broken down into these categories. So, while these categorical distinctions may make diagnosis easier and more expedient, they may not always lead to the correct diagnosis. If the diagnosis is wrong, then the patient is unlikely to benefit from treatment—and this is the danger.

CATEGORIZING DEPRESSION

The problem with categorical distinctions is they are by no means reliable or easily determinable. One of the major debates that continues to flourish in the field of depression concerns the number and nature of different types of depression. Despite its frequent use by physicians and therapists as a diagnostic tool, this question of categorizing depression still remains controversial, conflicting, and unresolved.

Kraepelin in 1921 (see Gold, 1995) conceptualized all depressive symptoms as one illness, referred to as manic-depressive psychosis. However, since Kraepelin's time, controversies and conflicts have abounded about whether or not depression could be or even should be broken down in terms of different types and subtypes, whether or not they formed part of a continuum from the normal personality, or whether they are even diseases at all. Current research trends tend to indicate that depression has different types and subtypes, although the nature and number of these categories are themselves controversial and far from clear. In fact, there are likely many types and subtypes of depressive illness that have not as yet been identified.

General Problems in Categorizing Depression

Below, some of the different types and subtypes of depression are discussed, but first I consider more general problems in attempting to categorize depression at all. Many professionals, for example, find that these categories are helpful in diagnosing depression, while others ignore them entirely, so there is no consensus among health care professionals as to their validity or application.

In addition, there are cultural differences associated with the current classification system, which can also render diagnosis problematic. While the DSM remains a main source of diagnosis in the United States, the International Classification of Disease (ICD) is more influential in Europe and elsewhere but does not describe the symptoms and categories in the same way as the DSM. Thus, there is no professional uniformity in the way depression is conceptualized by clinicians and this can also lead to problems in diagnosis, particularly if the patient seeks help from more than one clinician.

Furthermore, depression offers a particularly unique problem because a whole host of conflicting and strongly held opinions about the disorder abound and diagnosing is not always an exact science. For example, one psychiatrist might emphasize the importance of the distinction between endogenous and reactive depression, while it will be of little use to another. The subjective nature of diagnosis also points to other cultural differences in interpreting symptoms. Intra- and intercultural differences in defining and diagnosing depression have been noted elsewhere. According to one author (see Payer, 1988), the stiff upper lip mentality that characterizes British society, for example, influences medical diagnosis and treatment. Since Britain "has little tolerance for individuals who fail to maintain their self-control," suggests the author, British physicians are more likely to label such people as sick in comparison with other countries. In terms of bipolar disorder, for example, psychiatrists in Britain are likely to diagnose such a patient as schizophrenic, emphasizing the manic symptoms.

Furthermore, in comparison with their French and German counterparts, British psychiatrists were seen as more likely to view unipolar and bipolar depression more broadly and diagnosed 23% of patients from a group bipolar compared with 14% of German psychiatrists and only 5% of the French.

Another major problem with classifying depression into category types is the tendency for some clinicians to try to "fit" or even force a patient's symptoms into the existing classifications. But depressive symptoms do not always easily fit nicely into little diagnostic checklists or boxes as Shelly's case exemplified.

UNIPOLAR AND BIPOLAR CATEGORIES OF DEPRESSION

One of the most important distinctions that is made in diagnosing depressive symptoms concerns the unipolar and bipolar distinction, and it is probably the first such distinction that clinicians make for diagnosis. While much of the evidence indicates that these are two distinct disorders and they are treated as such, again this distinction is by no means conclusive.

Unipolar Disorder

Unipolar symptoms usually refer to the melancholic symptoms of depression, described earlier, and comprise both major depression and dysthymia. The vast majority of people with depression are diagnosed as having episodic, unipolar depression and thus this form of the illness receives the most attention in the literature. DSM-IV characterizes unipolar depression into the following subtypes, but the distinctions between the different subtypes of unipolar depression are themselves not always clear and there is quite a lot of overlap between categories.

Major Depressive Episode

This subtype comprises those symptoms of depression, discussed above, that have been present for a minimum of 2 weeks. In particular, these include a depressed mood or a general loss of interest in addition to four other symptoms of depression. One of the key words here is *episode*, because this type of depression is seen to be cyclical, episodic, and interspersed with periods of normal mental health.

Dysthymic Disorder

This subtype is a fairly new category of depression replacing what was once referred to as *neurotic depression* and is sometimes referred to as *minor depression* or *chronic depression*. Dysthymia is characterized by a depressed mood that has persisted for the most part for at least 2 years. However, while these symptoms must be evident during this time frame, they are not seen as severe enough for a diagnosis of major depression, and because dysthymia is not viewed as episodic, it is not relieved by periods of normal mental health.

People with dysthymia complain of feeling sad or down. In addition, during the depressed mood periods, increased or decreased sleep patterns, lack of energy and increased fatigue, low self-esteem, poor concentration and problems with decision-making and feelings of despair are also evident. Individuals may also describe lack of interest and be self-critical, often describing themselves as dull, uninteresting, or incapable. Because these symptoms persist and become very much a part of the person's daily experience, they are often seen as ingrained into the personality, a sort of "I have always been this way" attitude, and in fact may not even be reported unless probed by the interviewer. Furthermore, dysthymics may be both chronically depressed and also suffer from episodic depression.

Depressive Disorder Not Otherwise Specified

This subtype describes depressive symptoms that are different from those of other types of depression. These include certain syndromes related to premenstrual problems, minor depressive episodes, typified when the individual has fewer symptoms of depression than would meet the requirement for a major depressive episode, but still in evidence for at least 2 weeks, recurrent brief depressive disorder, which describes episodes of depression that last for at least 2 days and up to 2 weeks, not connected to the menstrual cycle and occurring at least once a month for a year, and psychotic symptoms associated with schizophrenia.

Psychotic Depressive Disorder of Schizophrenia

This subtype describes a major depressive episode that occurs during the residual phase of schizophrenia.

Other Situations

In this subtype the patient has been diagnosed as having a depressive disorder but the clinician is unable to determine whether the symptoms are related to a medical condition or substance abuse.

Bipolar Disorder

The other type of depressive illness, *bipolar disorder*, or *manic depression* as it was once called, tends to receive less attention than its unipolar counterpart, largely because it affects fewer people. Only about 5 to 10% of people with depression are diagnosed with bipolar disorder. It is thought that bipolar depression, the cause of which is believed to be genetic, may be the result of low levels of neurotransmitters, while the symptoms of mania are associated with excessively high levels of these chemicals. Symptoms of mania (Table 15), described in more detail below, can also occur alone, but this is very uncommon.

In addition to the melancholic symptoms of unipolar depression, those with bipolar depression also experience alternating epi-

Table 15. Symptoms of Mania

Psychological symptoms	Physical symptoms
Euphoric mood	Rapid speech
Flight of ideas	Reduced need for sleep
Heightened self-esteem	Excessive appetite
Delusions and grandiose thoughts	Restlessness
Impulsive behavior	
Impaired judgment	
Excessive uninhibited behavior	
Irritability	
Distracted	
Reckless behavior—spending, gambling	

sodes of mania, noted in Table 15. The defining features of a manic episode are a distinct period during which there is an unusually hyperactive, elevated, irritable, or expansive mood, which must persist for at least 1 week. There is sometimes the misconception that mania is always associated with a heightened or elevated mood, but this need not be the case. In addition, there must be signs of at least three other symptoms including an inflated sense of self-esteem or grandiosity, a reduction in required sleep, flight of ideas or racing thoughts, increased distraction, psychomotor agitation, increased attention to goal-directed ideas or plans, and excessive pleasure seeking which can lead to painful consequences. Often these disturbances must be quite severe and extreme enough to cause problems in social or occupational roles and sometimes can require hospitalization if hallucinations and delusions are also present. However, the mood episode must not be the result of the physiological effects of drug abuse or medication or exposure to other toxins or electroshock therapy for depression or be the result of other physiological effects of a general medical condition like multiple sclerosis.

The elevated mood state associated with a manic episode can be described as euphoric, cheerful, or high. Although this elevated mood may initially be viewed as infectious by those around the individual, it is soon seen as excessive. Expansive moods can be seen as those involving incessant and overtly enthusiastic desires for sexual, occupational, or interpersonal interactions. (A psychiatrist colleague of mine, discussing a bipolar depression patient of his, related that he can always tell when she is entering a manic phase, because her libido increases, which in evident by her increasingly shorter hemlines!) In this way, such a person may start engaging in prolonged chats with strangers. While symptoms of elevated mood are considered the main feature of mania, irritability may be the more predominant mood disturbance. The alternation between euphoria and irritability or lability of mood is frequently obvious.

There is also a tendency for the individual to present symptoms of an inflated self-esteem, which ranges from the uncritical self-confident to extreme grandiosity, which may even reach delusional proportions. These individuals may offer their advice on matters they know little about—how to solve world poverty—or despite their lack of talent, may start to write a novel or seek publicity for an invention. Grandiose delusions are particularly frequent, including having a special relationship with God, other religious figures, or prominent politicians.

In addition, there is usually, almost always, a decreased need for sleep. The manic individual typically wakes up after only a few hours of sleep, full of energy. Sometimes the person can go days without sleep and not feel the effects of fatigue.

Speech patterns are also noticeable. The voice becomes loud, rapid, difficult to interrupt. Such people may talk endlessly for hours, not giving others any opportunity to respond. They may become theatrical, overdramatic, sometimes even singing. However, if the bipolar person's mood is irritable, his or her speech may be full of complaints, hostile comment, and angry outbursts.

The individual's thoughts may also race at quite a fast pace; sometimes the mind works faster than the words can be articulated. Commonly there is a flight of ideas that is manifested by a monologue of accelerated speech, during which there are abrupt changes in conversation.

Manic individuals are often easily distracted. Sometimes it is difficult for them to screen out irrelevant objects, background conversations, or even furnishings in a room. In addition, they may have problems differentiating between thoughts that are relevant and irrelevant to a particular conversation.

There is a flurry in goal-directed activity that often involves excessive planning and participation in numerous activities. Increased sexual desire, fantasies, and behavior are apparent and these individuals may take on new business ventures, without regard to risk or to completing the venture sufficiently. This expansive thought, optimism that is often unwarranted, grandiosity, and poor judgment can often lead to spending sprees, reckless driving, and foolish business enterprises with disastrous consequences. Such a person may buy several houses without money to pay for them.

Moods may shift easily from anger to depression and the depressive and manic symptoms can occur simultaneously and may manifest themselves in several different ways, as follows.

A *mixed episode* is diagnosed when it occurs for at least 1 week, in which the criteria for both a manic episode and a major depressive episode are met almost daily. This individual shows symptoms of rapidly changing moods, sadness, euphoria, irritability, which are accompanied by other symptoms including sleep disturbances, agitation, irritability, problems with appetite, psychosis, and suicidal thinking. These disturbances must be sufficient to result in social or occupational difficulties and may even require hospitalization.

A *hypomanic* episode is characterized by a distinct period during which there is an abnormal and persistent elevated, expansive, or irritable mood that persists for at least 4 days. This abnormal mood state must also show at least three other symptoms including an inflated self-esteem or grandiosity, less sleep, flight of ideas, distractibility, rapid speech, and increased involvement in pleasure-seeking activities that have a high potential for disastrous consequences. The list of symptoms is identical to those for a manic episode, except that delusions or hallucinations cannot be present. Also in contrast to a manic episode, hypomania is not severe enough to cause a marked impairment in social or occupational performance or to require hospitalization. For some, the change in functioning might actually lead to an increase in efficiency, accomplishments, or creativity.

Symptoms such as these, however, may also be the result of antidepressant medication, electroconvulsive shock therapy, light therapy, or other medication prescribed for a medical problem.

As with unipolar depression, there are several different subtypes of bipolar disorder. DSM-IV categorizes the different forms of bipolar depression as follows.

Bipolar I Disorder

This subtype includes those symptoms of depression that involve at least one manic or mixed episode and in which episodes of depression are also present. The essential feature of bipolar I disorder is the occurrence of one or more manic or mixed episodes. Frequently, these individuals also have had one or more major depressive episodes. However, episodes of substance-induced mood disorder, related to the effects of medication, other treatments of depression, drug abuse, or exposure to a toxin, or related to another medical condition do not signal bipolar I depression.

Bipolar II Disorder

This subtype describes those symptoms of depression that include at least one episode of major depression and one or more episodes of hypomania, a less extreme form of mania. These individuals may not view their symptoms of hypomania as pathological, although others may describe this behavior as disturbed. The essential symptoms of bipolar II are the occurrence of one or more major depressive episodes accompanied by at least one hypomanic episode. Frequently, many patients, particularly those in the midst of a major depressive episode, may not even remember bouts of hypomania unless reminded and this information is crucial for the diagnosis of bipolar II.

Cyclothymia

This subtype, the bipolar equivalent of dysthymia, is diagnosed when the individual has persistent and chronic symptoms of hypomania which can be distinguished from a manic episode and episodes of depressive symptoms that do not meet the criteria for major depression.

Cyclothymia is diagnosed when an individual has persistent periods of both depression and hypomania. These bouts may be combined with, alternate, or intersperse with a period of normal mood for as much as 2 months. Cyclothymics show paired symptoms that are extreme. When depressed they avoid people, and when hypomanic they seek out company. When depressed they suffer from low self-esteem, and when hypomanic they believe they can accomplish anything. Such patients may also suffer major depressive and manic episodes. Thus, cyclothymia, like dysthymia, is not always so easily clinically defined.

Bipolar Disorder Not Otherwise Specified

This subtype describes those symptoms that do not match the criteria for any specific bipolar disorder or those symptoms for which there in inadequate or vague information. Symptoms typically include a very quick fluctuation, usually over days, between manic and depressive symptoms that do not meet the minimal duration criteria for either a manic or a major depressive episode, or persistent and recurrent hypomanic episodes without interconnected depressive symptoms, or situations in which the clinician has diagnosed bipolar disorder but is unable to detect a general medical condition or substance abuse as its cause.

While the unipolar and bipolar categories can provide a good basis for diagnosing depression and serve as useful guidelines, there are also certain limitations that require clarification. Overrelying on these categorical distinctions may lead clinicians to ignore other potentially valuable clues and symptoms. Shelly, for example, suffered terribly from mood swings during the worst phases of her depression and probably should have been diagnosed as having mixed episodes, because of their frequency and severity, when in fact even the existence of these mood swings was entirely ignored by physicians and psychotherapists.

Also, there is a potential danger that these categories can lead to labeling and stereotyping individuals with certain types of depression and this can be destructive to the patient's self-esteem, particularly if the diagnosis is not accurate. There is a further problem that needs to be addressed: insurance companies. Many insurance companies will not provide medical coverage to policy holders if they have a preexisting condition, like depression. Although this is a problem many Americans face, more and more British citizens are also taking out private medical coverage. A diagnosis of depression, particularly bipolar, is likely to present difficulties. One of my clients was wrongly diagnosed with a bipolar disorder, when he was actually suffering from an allergy to wheat. However, despite finding out the true cause of his mood swings, the original diagnosis stubbornly remained on his medical records, rendering future coverage almost impossible.

Other mimickers of bipolar disorder include low blood pressure, which ordinarily tends not to be considered a health disorder. For example, one study revealed that patients who had been diagnosed with bipolar disorder based on their symptoms, which included, among others, unreliability, problems with waking up in the morning, fatigue, irritability, melancholy, and mood swings, were actually suffering from low blood pressure.

Evaluating the Distinctions between Unipolar and Bipolar Depression

Although the distinction between unipolar and bipolar types of depression is used in diagnosis, it is still uncertain to what extent the distinction exists, if at all. There are several theories regarding the relationship between unipolar and bipolar disorders and the most accepted hypothesis to date is that they represent two distinct orders, but again, this view is by no means conclusive.

Unipolar and bipolar mood disorders do not seem to differ too much in terms of the quality of emotional health, and, in fact, they are quite similar. However, as presented in Table 16, there are some recognizable differences between them that indicate they are likely to be separate illnesses.

When bipolar patients are depressed, for example, they are usually more lethargic and tend to sleep more, while unipolar patients are more irritable and sleep less. The age of onset for bipolar is usually younger than that for unipolar and can first manifest itself even in adolescence. More first-degree relatives, typically parents and siblings, of bipolar patients suffer from both types of depression than do relatives of unipolar patients, and lithium carbonate has better therapeutic powers for bipolar patients when suffering a bout of depression than for unipolar.

Criticisms of the Unipolar–Bipolar Distinction

Direct comparisons between unipolar and bipolar patients are difficult to make, however, for several reasons. People with unipolar depression are more numerous and as a result are more likely to be a diverse collection of individuals when compared with their bipolar counterparts. In addition, bipolar patients can simultaneously suffer

Table 16. Comparisons of Unipolar and Bipolar Depression

Symptom	Unipolar	Bipolar
Age of onset	Thirty to forty	Twenties
Gender	Mostly women	Equal
Genetics	High risk if parents and siblings are diagnosed	High risk for both types of depression
Motor activity when depressed	Agitated	Lethargic
Sleep	Sleeps less	Sleeps more
Drug treatment	Tricyclics/heterocyclics	Lithium

from symptoms of both mania and depression or have them alternate for a period of days, while other individuals present only symptoms either of depression or of mania during an episode. So, people with bipolar depression can have symptoms of unipolar depression as well. Furthermore, research on the two disorders has shown that relatives of unipolar patients are at an increased risk for unipolar depression, whereas relatives of bipolar patients are at risk for both types, with a higher risk for unipolar. Perhaps, then, this information can support the argument that unipolar and bipolar disorders are not quite separate categories of depression, but rather represent different levels of severity of the some disorder. In this case, bipolar disorders would be seen as more severe.

ENDOGENOUS AND REACTIVE DEPRESSION

Another problem rests with the regularity with which physicians and nonmedical therapists diagnose and treat depression based on endogenous or reactive categories of the illness. In my view, the use of these two classifications for diagnostic and treatment purposes is excessive and can pose the most dangers to the patient.

Because depression can affect the individual with a variety of psychological and physical symptoms, it is often classified in terms of either biological (endogenous) or environmental (exogenous or reactive) factors. The word *endogenous* refers to from within the body; *exogenous* means coming from outside the body. This distinction also serves as the basis for psychiatric treatment of depression. These terms suggest that there are two distinct categories of depression, biological and psychological, and that the biological type is caused by some chemical malfunction, whereas the psychological type is triggered by some stressful life event.

This distinction has led to two main symptom clusters that are seen to aid diagnosis. Psychological depressions are seen to have more psychomotor retardation (slowness of movement), an inability to react to changes in the environment during depression, losing interest in life, and more physical symptoms. Endogenous depression is thought to show fewer of these symptoms, but early morning awakening, guilt, and suicidal behavior may be more associated with endogenous.

Traditionally, endogenous depression was considered the more serious and treated with antidepressant drugs. Reactive depression was thought to reflect an individual's inability to cope with life's problems and was treated almost exclusively with so-called "talk therapy." Now, however, with the advent of newer antidepressants, drugs can be prescribed for both types of depression.

Limitations of the Endogenous–Reactive Distinction

While it is feasible that depression could be caused by either internal or external factors alone, there are many problems with this categorical distinction, and anyone with depression should also be aware of them. First, there is no conclusive scientific evidence that proves that depression is caused mainly by either internal or external factors and, in fact, current research tends to focus on the psycho-biological interaction of depressive illness and the role of both the mind and body. Furthermore, because the symptoms of depression are the same, whatever the exact nature of the origins of the illness, it would be very difficult to determine whether or not the symptoms were caused by either internal or external factors. Moreover, clinicians tend to rely on patients' self-reports in determining the causes of depression. It is thought, for example, that reactive depression is caused by an inability to cope with life's problems. However, because people attempt to make sense of their lives when things go wrong and because the depressive illness distorts thought processes to such an extent that even pleasurable memories take on a bleak tone, people can so easily misattribute the cause of their depression to, say, recent unemployment or even more vaguely to problems at work. In addition, it has not been successfully proven that reactive depression is triggered more by stressful life events, and so-called endogenous symptoms of depression have been found to accompany stressful problems.

Thus, as a diagnostic tool, this distinction is unreliable. However, it still greatly influences how researchers and clinicians explain the causes of depression and develop and prescribe treatment strategies. Again, this can be a nightmare scenario in terms of diagnosis.

Seasonal Affective Disorder

Although there are problems with the reactive versus endogenous category of depression, this is not to say that biological subtypes of unipolar depression do not exist. At least two have been noted in the literature and there are probably many more. SAD is perhaps one of the most clear-cut forms of a biological subtype of episodic depression. It has been the focus of attention in recent years. SAD symptoms show a pattern of depression that first occurs in fall or winter and such individuals tend to overeat, crave carbohydrates, gain weight, and suffer from fatigue. This can be successfully treated with phototherapy, which involves exposing the patient to full-spectrum light. DSM-IV reports that both unipolar and bipolar disorders can be further subdiagnosed as seasonal, if there is a connection between an episode and a particular time of year. While the majority of studies on SAD have been conducted on people who experience depression in the winter months, other studies have shown that people can suffer symptoms of mania in the spring and summer (Rosenthal *et al.*, 1988). The most common explanations for this phenomenon link the mood disorders to changes in the length of daylight hours, and as a result, therapy for winter depressives involves exposing sufferers to bright white lights (Rosenthal *et al.*, 1988).

Postpartum Depression

Postpartum depression could also be viewed as a biological subtype of depression. Studies have shown that postnatal depression affects about 10% of new birth mothers. Yet, misconceptions about this type of depression abound. Sometimes postpartum depression is described as a type of psychosis, maternity blues, or is seen as the result of hormones or even as a woman's inability to function as a mother.

These conceptions about postpartum depression are myths. Maternity blues are best thought of as immediately succeeding the birth, when a woman's emotions are sometimes thrown into turmoil.

Most mothers experience this and in some respects it is viewed as normal and requires no treatment. Puerperal psychosis, by contrast, is a rare phenomenon, but has severe symptoms. Affecting about 1 in 500 new mothers, it is probably, like maternity blues set off by the biological readjustment that comes with childbirth, when hormones such as progesterone and estrogen that have increased substantially return to normal levels in a matter of a few days.

Puerperal psychosis requires treatment because it is a mental illness. In the majority of cases, major changes in emotions and in mood state are seen as the main symptoms, but sometimes irrational thoughts and disturbed senses are commonplace. For example, a new mother may imagine voices that want to threaten her or her baby and this can be quite a terrifying experience for her and her family. Puerperal psychoses often respond well to drug therapy and the mother is guaranteed of a complete recovery.

Postnatal depression is different. It is less severe than puerperal psychosis but is more common. It is also distinct from maternity blues because symptoms can appear within 1 or 2 months of delivery and can persist for several months without treatment. Symptoms include sleep disturbances, usually with fatigue, and the new mother can feel tense, blue, and irritable. She also loses interest in sex.

Postnatal depression often goes undetected and so untreated and its cause is still unknown. Generally, the disorder was attributed to being anxious about the new baby and an adjustment to a new routine. However, a recent breakthrough by scientists indicates that hormones might be the problem. British physicians have been successful in fighting postnatal depression with hormone replacement therapy. In clinical trials, women who started wearing HRT skin patches, which are normally reserved for menopausal women, reported an improvement in their condition and this treatment is offering hope. A low estrogen level is now thought to cause the disorder and since these patches contain the hormone estrogen, this discovery represents a major breakthrough.

PRIMARY AND SECONDARY DEPRESSION

As noted throughout this book, diagnosing the difference between primary and secondary depression is crucial in all cases of mood disorders and, in my view, is the most reliable category of depression.

The primary–secondary distinction separates depressive symptoms into two categories: symptoms that are indicative of mood disorders in their own right (primary) and those that are caused by some other medical disorder (secondary). However, while the evidence strongly supports the importance of this category in diagnosing depression, it is used less often and is overshadowed by the reliance on the unipolar–bipolar and endogenous–reactive categories of depression. This situation not only can be harmful to the patient, but also dangerous. Because depression can be the first symptom of a serious medical condition, it is first necessary to investigate the origins of the depressive symptoms to rule out any life-threatening illnesses.

It is obvious that clinical depression comes in many forms. But where the exact distinctions lie is anybody's guess and depends mainly on the personal prejudices of the practitioner. There is no uniformity or objective yardstick and this is a potential diagnostic nightmare. Clinical depression is a complex illness and manifests itself in many forms. However, just like the overreliance on behavioral symptoms, there is also a tendency for professionals to make a diagnosis based on certain types, subtypes, and categories of depression. Shelly's many symptoms, for example, did not fit neatly into any category.

In my view, then, researchers and health care professionals should begin conceptualizing depressive symptoms in the way specified in Table 17.

Table 17.   Categories of Depression Revised

	Unipolar disorder	Bipolar disorder
Primary depression	Single or recurrent episode	Mania or manic-depressive disorder

Secondary depression	Other psychiatric disorders
	  Alcoholism
	  Dementia
	  Schizophrenia
		Systemic medical illness
		  Central nervous system disorders
		  Drug-induced disorders
		  Infections
		  Endocrine disorders

Adapted from Gold (1995).

Part Two has examined some of the many problems related to current diagnostic practices for depression. Because of the tendency for researchers and health care professionals to rely on the outdated assumption that depression results from either a neurochemical breakdown or psychological problems, combined with practitioners' bias emphasizing the emotional symptoms of depression, diagnosis of the disorder tends to be rife with problems. It is thus not surprising that these limitations of the diagnostic process lead to problems in establishing effective treatments.

III

Evaluating Treatments
for Depression

Problems Related to Physiological Treatments

With major problems in explaining and diagnosing depression, it is obvious that flaws also exist in treating the illness, mostly because the prescribed treatments tend to fall rigidly along the lines of either physiological or psychological therapies and are recommended without laboratory tests confirming or ruling out depression.

In the Introduction, it was mentioned that as many as 90% of all depressed cases could be treated effectively. However, given the aforementioned limitations and flaws, it is not surprising that only about 20% of depressed people are seeking treatment, and, according to one study conducted by the National Institute of Mental Health (reported in Gold, 1995), among those who are treated for depression, only about 60% recovered after 6 months of treatment and only about a third of those reported being free of symptoms.

Throughout this book, many examples have been given of the ways in which academics, scientists, other researchers, and health care professionals have unsatisfactorily and inadequately attempted to explain many aspects of clinical depression, the symptoms, types and subtypes, vulnerability factors, the course of depression, and theories on the origins of the illness. There are many problems with the ways in which the illness is conceptualized and explained and conflicts about the nature of the mood disorder abound among the experts in the field. However, this lack of consensus is not just an academic issue. While scientists continue to argue among themselves about the different types and causes of depression, affected patients and clients are the ones who suffer the consequences.

SOME GENERAL LIMITATIONS OF TREATMENTS

First, it is human nature to try to make sense of our lives when things go wrong. Symptoms of depression, no matter what the cause, are often expressed psychologically and it is tempting to try to explain the pain by attributing it to a recent disappointment or personal tragedy. In Shelly's case, she just assumed that her depressive illness was a result of her being isolated in a new country. No doubt this contributed significantly to and helped to maintain her symptoms, but the worst symptoms were the result of an intolerance to coffee and sugar.

Thus, clinicians and physicians should never accept any client's symptoms at face value, tempting and logical though it may seem. With depression, they have to look beyond the seemingly obvious. And the only way to find out conclusively (or at best approximately) is by performing certain diagnostic tests.

Second, the treatment strategies offered mostly focus on the pathology of *either* the brain *or* the body, and as such tend to be divided along the endogenous–reactive lines. As previously discussed, scientists tend to view depression either as a neurochemical malfunction or as an inability of some people to cope with their problems. This conceptualization is shortsighted for several reasons, but mostly because it fails to account for the psychobiological nature of the illness and its many causes.

Third, scientists still do not fully understand how antidepressants work or why drugs have certain side effects.

Fourth, although experts now tend to agree that depression can be categorized into subtypes, they more often treat depression as one illness. Instead, we should be focusing more on the idea that certain therapies and treatments are more effective for certain kinds of depressive subtypes.

Fifth, treatments for depression tend to ignore the illness's high spontaneous remission rate. In the majority of cases, symptoms of depression resolve by themselves, without any form of drugs or therapy. So, while health care professionals may think the illness is relieved because of a particular type of therapy, the remission may in fact reflect the natural course of the disorder.

PHYSIOLOGICAL TREATMENTS

Medical doctors, usually psychiatrists, often prescribe certain physiological or somatic treatments to help depressed patients. These include antidepressant drugs and, to a lesser extent, electro-convulsive shock therapy. Drug therapies have several advantages. Most depressed patients can receive some timely benefit from drug therapies, which are quite economical in terms of cost, whereas psychological therapies can be time-consuming, expensive, and have no guarantee of any relief from symptoms.

Since it is reasonably conclusive at this stage that the neuro-transmitters norepinephrine, epinephrine, and serotonin (and no doubt others yet to be discovered) are involved in many cases of depression and that individuals who have reduced levels of these chemicals are prone to mood disorders, drugs that restore them back to normal levels are often prescribed. As already mentioned, the monoamine oxidase inhibitors (MAOIs) were the first antidepres-sants. Although effective in alleviating symptoms, they were soon found to have serious side effects, including high blood pressure and a harmful, sometimes lethal reaction when combined with certain foods like cheese, yogurt, wine, yeast breads, chocolate, and various fruits and nuts.

The tricyclics were then developed, which had the advantage of not producing those harmful reactions with food. These drugs in-cluded Elavil, Tofranil, imipramine, and amitriptyline, and they worked by blocking and suppressing the reabsorption or reuptake of serotonin and norepinephrine, resulting in increased levels of those neurotransmitters in the brain. Tricyclics are an effective form of treatment, and up to 80 to 90% of depressed people report a relief from symptoms after taking these drugs.

The Second-Generation Antidepressants

Often hailed as miracle or wonder drugs, the second-generation antidepressants are the heterocyclics. These are regarded as more effective because they work *selectively* by preventing the reabsorption of mainly one transmitter, usually serotonin. For this reason they are also called *selective serotonin reuptake inhibitors* (SSRIs). Because these drugs block the reuptake of serotonin, more of the neurotransmitter remains in the system.

Although the heterocyclics are effective, it is important to note that they are *not* more effective than the older drugs. The beneficial effects and advantages of the second-generation drugs are only that they work faster and have fewer side effects.

Prozac is one of the new generation of antidepressant drugs and because it has received so much media attention, it deserves special mention here. Although there were widespread accounts of people on Prozac committing suicide or attacking their partners or engaging in other violent acts, most of these reports were anecdotal and the FDA ruled that the drug was safe.

Millions of people are now prescribed Prozac (fluoxetine), Paxil (paroxetine HCl), and Zoloft (sertraline HCl), among others, which are recommended for a wide variety of other psychological problems, including eating disorders, anxiety, panic attacks, premenstrual tension, and obsessive-compulsive disorder.

Lithium

In the late 1940s, Australian psychiatrist John Cade noticed that lithium had antimanic properties and could be used to prevent mood swings. As a result of this discovery, lithium became the drug of choice to treat bipolar or manic-depression. Originally, lithium was prescribed to treat gout and as a substitute for salt to be used by patients with heart disease, but is no longer used for these purposes.

The discovery of the antimanic benefits of lithium revolutionized treatments for bipolar depression and it is now used to prevent relapse of both mania and depression in patients. It is also used when patients have mania alone and more recently has been used in combination with antidepressants to alleviate symptoms of depression that had been hard to treat. Although lithium cannot cure mania, it does seem to act as a powerful agent to prevent the onset of symptoms.

There are some problems with lithium, however. Because it may take as long as a year for some patients to receive the full benefits, many patients give up before it works. There are two main reasons why manic symptoms occur: patients failing to take lithium or the dosage of the drug being too low.

There are also side effects, some of which are quite toxic, such as stomach cramps, dehydration and excessive thirst, an increase in urine output, kidney problems, weight gain, nausea, an unusual metallic taste in the mouth, and thyroid problems.

The Side Effects of Antidepressants

Perhaps one day scientists will discover an antidepressant that will cure the pain and debilitating symptoms of depression without any complications; but for now, current drug therapies do unfortunately have certain side effects. All drugs have some kind of potential risks and those that treat depression are no exception. In fact, the MAOIs have been used in accidental and suicidal deaths. Fortunately, such incidents are rare, but there are some important side effects associated with antidepressants.

1. The downside of many drug therapies is that they do not work for everyone.
2. Determining the proper dosage is sometimes problematic, because each person metabolizes and responds to the drugs differently.
3. Antidepressants have some unpleasant side effects that can be as bothersome as the symptoms of depression. Additional medication may be required to remove or reduce those side effects.
4. Most drugs have some toxic properties and can harm the body, especially the liver.
5. Many drugs can lead to some form of dependency.
6. There is the further problem that drugs can interact with other medication the patient is taking, which can be serious or even fatal.

7. The drugs normally require anywhere from about 2 to 6 weeks to work, so suicidal patients must be monitored closely at this time.

Side Effects of Prozac

Although Prozac is hailed as a wonder drug and deemed safe for patient use for many kinds of psychiatric problems in addition to depression, there are still some side effects and potential side effects that should be of concern to any health professional involved in a depressed patient's treatment. They are:

1. Very few people have taken Prozac for more than 6 years, so we still do not know enough about long-term effects and ramifications of prolonged use.
2. Prozac patients often report experiencing wild and very vivid dreams and about one-third of people indicate problems such as insomnia or excessively frenetic dreams or nightmares.
3. More minor annoyances include gastrointestinal problems, headaches, and anxiousness.
4. We still do not know the effects of Prozac on pregnant women. As of now, there is no conclusive evidence that pregnant women on Prozac have a higher rate of birth defects, but there is always the chance that these defects might show up later, say in the form of a learning disability or a mood disorder. Also, it seems that there is an increased tendency, as with the other antidepressants, of miscarriage during the first trimester.
5. Sexual dysfunction has been associated with use of Prozac. A recent study reported that about one-third of Prozac patients experienced a decreased interest in sex. This can lead to problems in a relationship; however, loss of libido is one of the main symptoms of depression, so it is not necessarily a product of the drug.
6. More and more people relying on Prozac and similar antidepressants are at risk of developing a potentially lethal reaction known as the *serotonin syndrome*. If patients are

already taking a prescription drug, and then combine it with Prozac, they may be overloading their system with serotonin. Even some nonprescription drugs like certain cough medicines and diet pills can raise serotonin levels.

Some of the more common side effects associated with drug treatments for both unipolar and bipolar depression are summarized in Tables 18 and 19.

Because of the stigma that depression reflects a personal inadequacy or a moral weakness, many physicians believe that depressed individuals should face up to their problems and find solutions. For that reason, antidepressants are not prescribed, being seen instead as an easy escape. This negative attitude is as ill-informed as it is unhelpful. However, this view also indicates that the widespread myths about the illness survive. Depression is a painful illness, often a very debilitating one, and there is no reason for anyone to suffer needlessly from its severe and debilitating symptoms. After all, patients taking insulin for diabetes or antihistamines for allergies would never be challenged about the medication they take.

ELECTROCONVULSIVE SHOCK THERAPY

In addition to drug therapies, another form of physiological treatment is electroconvulsive shock therapy (ECT). Many people, even those who work with depressed patients and clients, are surprised to learn that ECT is still used to combat symptoms of depression. ECT certainly has a dubious reputation and its use remains both emotionally and politically controversial today, in part the result of its portrayal in such films as *One Flew Over the Cuckoo's Nest* and in such books as Sylvia Plath's *The Bell Jar* (1963).

In general, however, ECT is used only on people with severe depression who have not been treated successfully with drugs, or those who are not regarded as good candidates for antidepressants because of another existing medical condition. Also, because antidepressants can take a few weeks to work, ECT usually offers more immediate relief for those with severe depression and who are in danger of committing suicide.

Table 18. Some Side Effects
of Drug Therapies Used
in Treating Unipolar Depression

Drug type
  Monoamine oxidase inhibirors
    Nardil (phenelzine sulfate)
    Parnate (tranylcypromine sulfate)
  Tricyclics
    Adapin (doxepin HCl)
    Anafranil (clomipramine HCl)
    Elavil (amitriptyline)
    Norpramin (desipramine HCl)
    Pamelor (nortriptyline HCl)
    Pertofrane (desipramine HCl)
    Sinequan (doxepin HCl)
    Surmontil (trimipramine maleate)
    Tofranil (imipramine HCl)
    Vivactil (protriptyline HCl)
  Second generation: unipolar
    Asendin (amoxapine)
    Desyrel (trazodone HCl)
    Effexor (venlafaxine HCl)
    Ludiomil (maprotiline HCl)
    Paxil (paroxetine HCl)
    Prozac (fluoxetine)
    Wellbutrin (bupropion HCl)
    Zoloft (sertraline HCl)
Side effects
  Potentially fatal high blood pressure
  Dizziness
  Headache
  Nausea
  Dry mouth
  Fatal overdose
  Heart attack, stroke
  Hypotension
  Blurry vision
  Fatigue
  Anxiety
  Gastrointestinal complaints
  Dry mouth
  Sexual dysfunction
  Weight gain
  Nervousness
  Fatigue
  Gastrointestinal complaints
  Dizziness
  Headache

Table 19. Side Effects of Drug Treatments
for Bipolar Depression

Drug	Side effects
Lithium	Tremors
	Gastrointestinal problems
	Coordination problems
	Dizziness
	Cardiac arrhythmia
	Blurry vision
	Tiredness
Bupropion (Wellbutrin)	Agitation
	Dry mouth
	Insomnia
	Headache
	Gastrointestinal problems
	Tremors
	Seizures
	Weight loss

In ECT, a current is sent to the brain so as to induce a seizure and temporary unconsciousness. The seizure is seen as central to the treatment. Previously electrodes were placed on both sides of the brain (bilateral), but now unilateral ECT, on one side of the brain, is more commonly used. In the past, people often tore muscles or fractured bones during ECT treatment. Nowadays, however, the patient is given muscle relaxants and is asleep during the treatment, and is constantly checked for vital signs. However, there are some obvious disadvantages with ECT therapy. Prolonged and continued use may cause brain damage and can lead to permanent or temporary memory impairments.

The history of ECT is interesting and worth mentioning, not least of which because it helps to illustrate the accidental and random way in which scientific discoveries are made. In the early part of this century, a physician named von Meduna observed that psychotic patients who also suffered from epilepsy made improvements following an attack. He believed that the excessive neural activity in the brain, as a result of the epileptic seizure, somehow led to improvements in the patient's mental state. Sometime later, in the 1930s, an Italian psychiatrist, Ugo Cerletti, developed a method for inducing seizures in patients. Based on his observations from a local slaughterhouse, where jolts of electricity were applied to the animal's head to stun them before they were killed, it was thought that the electric current produced a seizure that resembled an epileptic fit. Cerletti had hoped to use electricity to induce a safe seizure and as a result of much experimentation, ECT arrived and became a form of treatment. Although it was originally used to treat a wide variety of mental health problems, including schizophrenia, it is now used exclusively for depression.

The best ECT candidates among depressed patients are:

- Patients who have previously responded well to ECT
- Patients with severe psychotic symptoms of depression
- Patients who are at serious risk of suicide
- Patients who are unable to take antidepressants
- Patients whose symptoms are not alleviated by antidepressants
- Elderly patients (ECT is seen as a safer alternative to antidepressants)

ANTIDEPRESSANT TREATMENTS CURRENTLY UNDER DEVELOPMENT

Electromagnetic Device

As previously mentioned, research into the biological and physiological causes of depression continues to thrive, and scientists and health care professionals of all descriptions should be encouraged by reports of new forms of treatment for depression. One interesting, but alternative, approach to treatment that is still very much in the development stage is a hand-held electromagnetic device. This device can be applied to a specific part of the brain and stimulates brain tissue in a more precise manner than ECT, while not inducing seizures or convulsions.

The device is held by a physician against the head of a depressed patient for about half an hour every other day. The baseball glove-sized device emits pulses of a magnetic field barely detectable by the patient, and this seems to help some patients escape their depression.

Mark George and his colleagues at the National Institute of Mental Health (*New Scientist*, July 1995) believe that while this is not a total cure, magnetic impulses seem to alleviate symptoms by temporarily resetting the brain. But this is still in the research stages. Some people reported feeling happy for the first time in years. The treatment is applied to the left side of the head and has produced no ill effects.

While this treatment strategy has not been perfected, at least it represents a potential future therapy that may be particularly beneficial to people who do not benefit from antidepressants or ECT.

Saint-John's-Wort

Herbalists and others have long recognized the soothing and calming properties of Saint-John's-Wort and now pharmacologists in Germany are conducting trials of the extract from this plant as a rival to chemical antidepressants. Clinicians are particularly hopeful about this herb because the side effects are minimal. In addition to relieving symptoms of depression, Saint-John's-Wort is also useful in alleviating anxiety.

In summary, this chapter has considered some physiological treatments for depression, including antidepressants, electroshock therapy, and alternative therapies. When based on a proper diagnosis, such treatments can be effective, although there are concerns about side effects, long-term safety, and receiving the appropriate drug dosage. However, physiological therapies are only part of a treatment program. Psychological therapies are also prescribed.

11

Problems Related to Psychological Treatments

Because the symptoms of depression are often interpreted as an emotional disorder, a wide variety of psychological therapies are available. With so much research into the biological causes of depression and the availability of physiological antidepressant treatments, it might be tempting to question the relevance of talk therapy. While I remain encouraged that the physical aspects of depressive illness are gaining a greater degree of acceptance, it is also essential to analyze the current trends in psychological therapies, because they are still an influential treatment form.

This stated, however, an earlier chapter considered the flaws found in many of the psychological theories of depression and, logically, the therapies based on these theories are also limited. The aim of this chapter is to examine these therapies in more detail. However, before beginning that discussion, some general problems that are applicable to all of the different therapies are introduced.

GENERAL LIMITATIONS OF PSYCHOLOGICAL TREATMENTS

First, many psychologists, counselors, and other therapists fail to advise their clients to obtain a thorough medical examination and proper diagnosis of depression, this failure upholding the myth that depressive illness is an emotional disorder. As a result, clients are likely to begin a course of therapy, which could take several months or years, for an illness they may not have.

Second, many of these theories are outdated, anachronistic, and fail to keep up with recent discoveries related to the physiology of depression—and thus perpetuate the mind–body distinction.

Third, since therapists make presumptions about human behavior and depression, and have a tendency to blame clients for their symptoms, they often instill in individuals neurotic impulses that were not present before treatment. For example, a client of mine, Ellen, was treated for anorexia and depression. Her previous therapist kept stressing that her symptoms of mood and eating disorders were the result of her parents' marital breakup when she was 3. Ellen does not remember much about her father, having been raised by her mother in what she described as a "warm, loving home." Although feelings of abandonment could have been the cause of her symptoms, Ellen's therapist ignored the link between anorexia, depression, and low levels of serotonin. The abnormally low levels of this neurotransmitter are more likely the cause of her illnesses.

Fourth, these therapies tend to ignore the needs of depressed patients. Since many psychological therapies aim to identify the reasons why a patient has developed depression, they usually focus on the client's childhood, traumatic experiences, and relationships with the parents. However, this investigation into the client's personal "archaeology" is neither logical nor practical. In the first instance, because all memories, even the happiest ones, tend to be impaired when someone is depressed, isolating the exact trigger is likely to be time-consuming, if not impossible.

Instead, depressed patients need and prefer practical strategies to help them cope with their symptoms and to find effective treatments irrespective of their cause.

Fifth, there are many different types of therapists, all of whom have different levels of training and education, so there is a lack of consensus among psychological therapists as to the best way to treat depression.

Sixth, some therapies were not designed to treat depression, while others are actually dangerous for depressed patients.

Seventh, not only do these therapies stress that depression is an emotional illness, they also tend to focus on a particular psychological symptom that they assume is the problem. Therefore, these therapies tend to treat symptoms, not the causes of depression, and because they focus on one symptom, they ignore the others.

Eighth, therapists try to force fit client's problems and symptoms into their preferred treatment strategy, whether or not appropriate for that particular case. This is generally because each therapist and clinical psychologist was trained in and adopted a particular approach to therapy. So, their methods of treating problems such as depression largely depend on their school's or institute's training program.

While Shelly's disastrous encounters with therapists were the subject of an earlier chapter the experiences of another client, Michelle, also illustrate this point. One evening several years ago, Michelle was attacked, and while she managed to escape unhurt, it was nonetheless a particularly frightening experience. A few days after the event, Michelle developed symptoms of anxiety and distress, and was clearly showing other symptoms of posttraumatic stress disorder. Also at that time, she was doing her best to cope with her symptoms of depression, and until this incident she was emotionally stable. Michelle was understandably very concerned that this attack might trigger an episode of depression, particularly because her emotional stability at that time was fragile.

Michelle sought help from a clinical psychologist who had been recommended by her physician. She recounted to the therapist the details of the attack, the delayed onset of symptoms of distress, and her chronic problems with depression. The woman, however, ignored everything Michelle told her except for the words *victim* and *victimization*. Now, it was pretty obvious that Michelle had been just one of a great many other victims of crimes that occur everyday, for which the word *victim* is commonly used when we talk about crime. However, the therapist kept focusing on Michelle's self-perceptions of being a victim and attempted to probe her early childhood memories to find the root cause of this "victimization." One hour and £50 later, Michelle was still trying to convince the therapist that, her other problems aside, the reason for the present visit related to the aftereffects of the attack. Michelle's therapist remained unconvinced. Instead, she insisted that all of Michelle's problems stemmed from her negative self-view of victimization.

After the session ended, Michelle left and never returned. A few days later, her symptoms of distress disappeared and she felt fine again.

Michelle's experience with the therapist should be a source of concern for health care professionals treating clients, especially because her situation is not unique. It may seem obvious, but in order for therapists to provide the most effective help and support for their clients, they should not impose their theoretical framework in assessing and treating clients. With depressed clients, in particular, it would be helpful for therapists to have an in-depth understanding of all of the advantages, disadvantages, merits, and limitations of the various psychological treatments available.

PSYCHOANALYSIS

One of the main psychotherapeutic treatments for depression is psychoanalysis, based on the theories discussed in the previous section. Briefly, the main traditional goal of psychoanalysis is to make conscious to the client those impulses and conflicts that are buried deep within the subconscious mind. In other words, the aim is to make the unconscious conscious. Through this process, the client can reexperience—in a safe context—repressed feelings and wishes that have been the source of frustration in childhood.

In order to achieve this goal, the analyst or therapist reflects back or "mirrors" to the client exactly what he or she says and in this way actively interprets the significance of what the client is reporting. The process by which the client gains—through the therapist's interpretations—insight into his or her unconscious conflicts causing disturbances and problems is known as *working through*. The techniques commonly used to achieve this goal are called *free associations*, *resistance*, *dreams*, and *transference*.

The analysis of free associations has been the predominant psychoanalytic technique used. In this process, the client is encouraged to reveal all thoughts and feelings that come into mind, even those that seem strange, trivial, insignificant, irrelevant, and embarrassing. According to Freud, free association is essential to unlocking meaningful information.

Another central technique of psychoanalysis is that of analysis of resistance, and here the therapist charts the client's behaviors that block his or her progress. Indicators of resistance include, for example, a client's tendency to mention important matters just before the end of the therapy session, his or her tendency to spend a lot of time discussing trivial topics, wasting time, acting in a difficult or belligerent manner, arriving for the appointment late, missing sessions, and changing the subject.

By identifying and interpreting the meaning of these resistant tendencies, the therapist hopes to assist the individual client to discover the unconscious conflicts that are at their core. For example, if a client tries to change the topic every time the therapist mentions a relationship with his or her mother, the analyst will likely interpret this as an unconscious emotional conflict with the mother.

Freud also held that the analysis of dreams was the pathway to the unconscious because it is here that unconscious sexual and aggressive conflicts reveal themselves.

While these techniques are important in this process, the essential factor in psychoanalysis is the analysis of transference. Transference refers to the client's tendency to treat the therapist as he or she would treat other important people in everyday life, including a partner, parent, or boss. Transference can be either negative or positive. With positive transference, the client behaves in an approving and affectionate manner toward the therapist. With negative transference, in contrast, the client is disapproving, rejecting, and critical. Through the process of transference, the therapist hopes to assist the client in gaining important insight into the origins of the emotional distress and difficulties.

In classical psychoanalysis, the analyst is supposed to remain essentially anonymous in that he or she should not demonstrate any emotion, reveal any personal information, and not make value judgments about anything the client says or does. Normally, but not always, the client lies down on the couch and the analyst traditionally sits behind the client, out of his or her sight line. The therapist's role is to be an "ambiguous object" onto whom the client can project feelings. But there should also be a good, constructive working relationship.

Freudian psychoanalysis has sprouted several different variations. Jung and Adler, who originally were colleagues of Freud's, before going out on their own, and later, neo-Freudians, who were not Freud's students, such as Karen Horney, Melanie Klein, Erich Fromm, and Jacques Lacan, all devised their own versions of analysis.

In the 1950s, psychoanalysis was the most popular form of analysis, but it is much more rarely used today. There are several drawbacks associated with psychoanalysis, one being that it is a long-term treatment strategy, which can be expensive. In many cases, the client is expected to attend therapy several times a week, which can span many years, even decades. Further, there is no guarantee of relief from symptoms or even a cure. More importantly, even Freud believed that depression *was not* a suitable illness for psychoanalysis.

To overcome many of these problems with traditional psychoanalysis, the trend today is to employ what is commonly called *psychodynamic therapy*, which adopts some of the strategies of psychoanalysis, but with treatment lasting months instead of years. Psychodynamic therapists seek out information on past and present relationships instead of trying to discover unconscious conflicts.

THE BEHAVIORAL THERAPIES

This type of therapy links thoughts and actions. When people have acquired a new way of thinking, they usually adopt a corresponding behavior pattern. So, if people learn to change maladaptive thoughts, their behavior will change too. And, since behaving in a healthier way makes people feel better, they continue to act in this newer, more beneficial way—according to this theory.

The late Hans Eysenck, one of the world's most famous psychologists, coined the term *behavior therapy* to describe those psychological treatment strategies that aim to change a person's maladaptive behavior rather than delve into the individual's unconscious mind to discover hidden conflicts. He argued that just because an individual knows that he or she is depressed and can experience some form of cathartic release, which is the aim of psychoanalysis, does not guarantee that the client will become less depressed. For example, people may know it is silly to be afraid of a little, harmless spider, but it does not stop them from screaming when they see one. So, in contrast to the traditional psychoanalytic approach, the behavioral tradition dismisses the notion or the importance of the subconscious mind and hidden conflicts and instead stresses the individual's current, but maladaptive behavior patterns.

Operant Conditioning

One strategy behavioral therapists often use is called *operant conditioning*, which can be useful for treating some symptoms of depression. Operant conditioning treatments aim to change maladaptive behavior patterns by controlling the outcomes. This is more popularly known as *behavior modification*, based on the work of B. F. Skinner. The most widespread forms of behavior modification rely on positive reinforcement. Positive reinforcement is sometimes referred to as the *token economy*, in which good behavior is rewarded so as to reinforce desired behaviors, the reward later being applied to privileges. For example, a therapist typically would encourage a client to reward him- or herself for taking the initiative in a conversation, making a telephone inquiry about a job advertisement, or setting up an interview. By being rewarded for the task, the client should feel better about him- or herself and gain confidence and self-esteem.

Social Learning

Social learning therapy is another popular technique of behavioral therapists and can benefit depressed clients. Here, they would typically instruct their clients to observe other people, either in person or on videotape, who have adaptive, healthy behaviors. The philosophy here is that clients are able to learn and model good social skills or to overcome fears by watching how others behave in certain situations and copying them. Alternatively, the therapist may model the desired behavior while the client observes. This can be a particularly successful strategy that helps people gain confidence through developing more effective social skills.

This is a short-term treatment strategy and the assumption of therapists is that the client should be cured in months, not years, so that behavioral therapy is preferable to psychoanalysis and psychodynamic therapy. This stated, however, it assumes that the cause of depression is maladaptive behavior patterns that can be unlearned and replaced with healthy ones. Although I applaud the use of

practical strategies to encourage confidence and self-esteem, therapists should be reminded that feelings of insecurity and a desire for
social withdrawal are cardinal symptoms of depression, not the
causes.

INTERPERSONAL THERAPY

Another related short-term treatment strategy is interpersonal
therapy. Since depressed people live in a social world, relationships
are also likely to be affected when someone becomes depressed.
Partners, children, employers, parents, colleagues, and friends can
also be subjected to the disruptive and dysfunctional nature of this
mood disorder, including social withdrawal, irritability, and mood
swings.

Interpersonal therapy was developed by Klerman and Weiss-
man who devised guidelines for a short-term type of therapy that
assists clients in acknowledging, discovering, and dealing with their
current problems with other people, and this therapy has also been
seen as successful in helping depressed people. To interpersonal
therapists, it is of little importance whether the troubled relationship
is the root cause or the result of depression. Instead, they focus on the
nature of the dysfunctional relationship and aim to help the client
resolve it, usually through role-playing.

In addition, this type of therapy aims to help someone suffering
from social withdrawal develop and build confidence and some self-
esteem and the social skills to build relationships with other people
and/or repair current ones.

COGNITIVE THERAPY

Cognitive therapy is probably the most widespread and influential form of therapy for depression today. As previously discussed,
cognitive therapists argue that events in themselves do not cause
maladaptive emotions or behaviors, but rather it is our interpretation
of the events that does so. Chapter Five considered Dr. Beck's assumption that depression is the result of negative beliefs about oneself, the world, and the future, which is the negative triad. Because
depressed people tend to blame themselves rather than circum-

stances for their misfortunes, this therapy approach seeks to undo that type of thinking. According to cognitive therapists, changes in the way we think can give rise to irrational emotions and patterns of behavior that are maladaptive. For example, a student might claim that he fails exams because he is stupid and therefore will never find a job or be successful in life. The cognitive therapist would typically ask such a client why he thinks he is not performing well at school, proposing instead that poor study habits or not enough study time might be at fault. By identifying the real cause of the problem, the student then could adopt better study habits, improve grades and thus career options.

Rational Emotive Therapy

Rational emotive therapy (RET or REBT) is another form of cognitive therapy. Albert Ellis is credited with developing RET, which has proved widespread and popular. Its basic premise is the A-B-C theory of emotion. A is seen as an activating event, B is an irrational belief, and C is the emotional consequence. Ellis (1962) argues that most people hold the belief that A causes C, when in reality it is B that causes C. For example, a student fails an exam (A) and becomes depressed (C). Ellis would say that the depression is the result not of the failure but of an irrational belief (B) that you must be perfect. It is, in his view, the irrational belief, not the failure, that is the cause of the depressive symptoms. Table 20 presents some of the more widespread irrational beliefs that typify many clients' experiences.

During therapy sessions, Ellis himself tends to adopt a Socratic approach with his clients and he can often be harsh, even argumentative, in challenging his clients to supply evidence for their irrational thoughts. Although Ellis favors a confrontational style, many RET therapists adopt a more empathetic relationship with their clients. In challenging views like: "I am worthless. I am a disaster. Nothing ever goes right," they will offer counterexamples that contradict these overgeneralizations such as abilities the client is overlooking or discounting. The therapist also often instructs the client to watch out for private monologues with her- or himself and to isolate all patterns of thinking that contribute to depression. Next, the therapist is likely to instruct the client to ponder through these negative and

Table 20.   Ellis's Most Common Irrational Beliefs

1. It is of the utmost importance that an individual is loved or approved of by
    almost every other important person in his or her social world.
2. I must be competent and successful in just about everything I do if I am to
    consider myself worthwhile.
3. Some people are evil and wicked and should be severely punished for their
    behavior.
4. It is dire, devastating, and catastrophic when things are not how I want them
    to be.
5. People have little or no control over their lot in life and happiness is caused
    externally.
6. One should be concerned about and keep dwelling on the possibility of some-
    thing frightening and dangerous happening.
7. It is hard to face up to certain problems and responsiblities and much easier to
    avoid them instead.
8. I should depend on other people and need to rely on someone who is stronger.
9. My past history is the most important thing in determining my present behavior.
    Just because something in the past had a devastating effect, it will always have
    that same effect.
10. It is my responsibility to be very upset about the problems of other people.

irrational thought patterns to understand how they prevent more positive, realistic, and healthy interpretations that reflect the circumstance more accurately.

Despite its widespread use in treating depression, cognitive therapy again makes the presumption that the illness is categorically caused by irrational thoughts. In some cases, no doubt, people are depressed for these reasons alone; however, as concentration and mood disturbances are classic symptoms of depression, they should not be confused with the origins of the illness. Although many cognitive therapists regard irrational beliefs or faulty thoughts to be the cause of mood disorders (Beck himself argued that negative thoughts breed negative feelings), there is little evidence at this stage to support this view.

HUMANISTIC THERAPY

The different types of therapy mentioned above have helped many people find relief from their symptoms of depression and, depending on the reasons why individuals are depressed and their psychological expressions of the illness, they can provide assistance. However, some other therapy options are far from helpful and are likely to endanger the depressed patient. One of these is humanistic therapy, and, while humanistic oriented therapies can help a wide range of people with a diverse set of symptoms, they really should be avoided when treating depression.

This type of therapy stresses the individual's conscious state and the present, the here and now, so it is very different from the psychoanalytic tradition and its emphasis on buried conflicts and the past. Another aspect is its emphasis on an individual's interpretation and subjective accounts of his or her experiences, unlike the behavioral approach, which stresses experiences that are objective and environmental or external. Finally, this therapeutic view encourages the client to express emotion freely, which is different from the cognitive approach, which aims to point out and control an individual's emotional interpretations.

Client-centered therapy (CCT), or person-centered therapy, is the most well-known version of humanistic therapy. Carl Rogers, formerly a psychoanalyst and probably one of the most influential of modern psychotherapists, first devised this type of therapy in the 1950s as a response to the psychoanalytic tradition.

This is not a Socratic or confrontational type of therapy in the fashion of RET. Instead the CCT therapist uses nondirective therapeutic techniques and does not question any faulty thinking of the client. The goal is toward self-actualization and the therapist helps clients come to terms with their own problems by providing a supportive atmosphere in which to probe the different potential answers to their problems. In theory, then, the therapy's goal is to provide a warm, stable, safe, and secure climate. In such a setting, clients will feel comfortable and better able to reflect on their problems, helping them eventually to reach their goals. CCT holds that a psychological disorder is the result of a breakdown between the individual's public face and private person. The therapist, through this safe environment, tries to decrease this gap. Unconditional positive regard and accurate empathy are techniques used by the therapist, who is an active listener and reflects back the individual's feelings.

On the surface it might seem that CCT offers the depressed person a lot of sympathy and support. However, this is the worst kind of treatment strategy for someone with depression. First, although the therapists adopt an active *listening* role, many clients with depression find them detached, uninterested, aloof, even bored. Regarding their therapists as unsympathetic to their problems, clients tend to feel rejected and even more inadequate after they leave therapy. In fact, Shelly, who was treated by a client-centered counselor, often felt so much worse after each session that she would immediately develop symptoms of anxiety and panic. Also, since some of the symptoms of depression are excessive rumination and dwelling about the misery and bleakness of life and the future and because depressed people often see no end to their symptoms, the nonguidance approach of CCT just exacerbates those feelings. Depressed people need therapists who can help support and encourage them and actively guide them to improving their life, whether it is through more effective social skills or inspiring confidence to apply for a new job. Cognitive, interpersonal, and behavioral therapies are better suited to the needs of depressed people.

HOW EFFECTIVE IS THERAPY?

This chapter has reviewed some psychological treatments that are considered the most scientifically grounded and valid, but it is important to ask: Is therapy generally effective? A 1982 study (see Milligan & Clare, 1994) found, for example, that three-quarters of clients were satisfied with their experiences of therapy. This stated, a recent study as part of a National Health Service review found that counseling on its own is "useless." So, which is it?

Problems in Determining the Effectiveness of Therapy

Although the effectiveness of therapy for all kinds of psychiatric symptoms has been the subject of wide debate and evaluation, the answer is not so straightforward and remains elusive. There are many different types of therapists, including psychiatrists, psychologists, counselors, social workers, nurses, religious figures, and paraprofessionals among many others all of whom aim to treat depression. Because of the diversity of these various professionals, in particular the varying levels of education, qualification, and experience, therapies are often in conflict with each other, further rendering the task of determining the effectiveness of therapy as a general area of investigation impossible.

In fact, the terms *therapy* and *effectiveness* are open to wide interpretations. Does *effective* mean a fast cure, a steady rate of improvement, the application of coping skills, the development of confidence or self-esteem? Of equal importance, it is also necessary to specify very carefully the exact person who is determining the effectiveness of the therapeutic program. Is it the client's health care professional? the client? the insurance company? There are many important variables that must be taken into account before we can even begin thinking about determining the effectiveness of therapy.

As a result, depending on the type of therapy, the therapist, goals, and definitions of effectiveness, rates of effectiveness are likely to vary. This said, the current debate on the issue can best be traced back to the early 1950s, when Dr. Hans Eysenck attempted to assess its value by looking at the progress of individuals seeking help for anxiety and depression. He found that the majority of these people improved and this would seem to suggest that psychoanalysis was effective in most cases. However, even more importantly, Eysenck also discovered that the same percentage of his control subjects, or those individuals not undergoing psychoanalysis, improved or went into *spontaneous remission*, as he called it. It was his belief that other events in these individuals' lives helped them improve. So, in the end, he concluded that psychotherapy was ineffective.

Eysenck's negative evaluation of the effectiveness received substantial criticisms and since then, there have been numerous other attempts to assess the effectiveness of talk therapy. However, this is not easy to prove on a scientific basis, since effectiveness is difficult to define, let alone measure. The concept of effectiveness differs greatly according to the goals and orientations of each therapy. Should therapy aim to help people explore and discover hidden conflicts? alleviate personal anguish? build self-esteem? help build confidence? help the individual cope with depressive symptoms or cure them? exchange maladaptive social skills for more socially acceptable ones?

The evaluation of effectiveness will also depend on the therapeutic traditions of the therapy. A rational-emotive therapist would hope that his or her client not be too harsh in self-assessment and learn self-acceptance; a behavioral therapist, that the client learn more effective social skills; and a psychoanalyst, that the client develop some understanding of hidden childhood traumas from which he or she is ultimately released.

There are other problems in establishing the effectiveness of psychotherapy. One is that the term *psychological treatment* includes so many different forms of treatment. Some professionals believe that all forms of psychotherapy have some beneficial effect and that no one particular treatment is necessarily objectively better than another.

Another problem in assessing the effectiveness of psychotherapy is the lack of objectives to be studied. For example, the effectiveness of psychoanalysis is rarely studied by experimental psychologists because it is difficult to measure things like hidden conflicts. Behavioral therapy, with its more objective anxiety hierarchy, is easier to quantify and study.

Also, even when clients do improve, health care professionals cannot demonstrate that the therapy was responsible for the improvement. Other factors presumably might be at work, such as the individual's motivation to improve or the rapport between client and therapist. Most importantly, physicians and psychologists have to take account of the rate of spontaneous remission. Recall that symptoms of depression last for about 3 to 6 months. Individuals receiving therapy during this time period may attribute their return to mental health to the therapy, when it may just reflect the natural course of the illness.

Is Therapy Effective for Depression?

If there are problems in determining the effectiveness of talk therapies in general, is it equally difficult to determine their success rates for depression? No doubt if we asked cognitive, behavioral, interpersonal, psychodynamic, and humanist therapists, psychiatrists, and others, each would claim that theirs is the most effective therapy for depression. Nevertheless, a number of studies have shown that the various therapies are pretty much equally effective.

For example, the National Institute of Mental Health (Gold, 1995) conducted a 16-week study on the effectiveness of psychotherapy for over 200 severely depressed patients, subdivided into four groups. One group received cognitive therapy, another interpersonal therapy, the third the antidepressant imipramine, and the fourth a placebo drug and some very limited supportive assistance from a therapist. The study found that subjects in all of the groups improved. About half of the patients showed great improvement in each of the three active treatment groups and even about a third of the participants in the placebo group found relief from their symptoms. The report concludes that the three active therapies (cognitive, interpersonal, and drug) were all equally effective, although the medication alleviated the symptoms much more quickly.

A study conducted by the University of Minnesota also compared cognitive, interpersonal, and drug therapies to see which was more effective. Drug and talk therapies were found to be equally effective in terms of relieving symptoms of depression, but patients who had "couch therapy" were less likely to relapse when compared with those on antidepressants for the same amount of time.

These studies tend to confirm that some treatments for depression are effective, but they do not conclusively point to which ones are the *most* effective. The most effective treatment strategy for mood disorders depends on the reasons why a person is depressed and his or her needs. However, other important factors must be acknowledged.

While the very nature of depression seems to be episodic for most people, that is, they will eventually regain their mental health and relief from their symptoms, with no drug or psychological intervention at all, a study (Brown, 1979) that investigated the improvement and recovery rate of female clients with anxiety and depression found that the recovery rate was related to the occurrence of a positive event in their lives. Thus, just as a negative event can trigger symptoms of depression, a positive event can produce mental well-being. According to the authors of the report, these positive events include *the anchoring dimension*, in which the client feels a sense of security, a *fresh start*, where the individual begins to feel a sense of hopefulness that a particular conflict will be resolved—such as that from a new job, a new relationship, a change in behavior, or moving to a new home—and *relief* from a difficult situation, without the necessity of a fresh start.

Of equal importance is evaluating the methodological framework of the studies themselves. We know so little about the origins of depression, but it is likely that there are very many factors involved. Studies evaluating the effectiveness of psychotherapy rarely specify which subtypes of depression are being treated. Assessing the effectiveness of different therapies could thus be misleading based on this alone. For example, in a study of individuals whose depression is related to psychological factors, cognitive therapy may show a high effectiveness rating. Conversely, if the individuals were depressed for biological or other reasons, cognitive therapy might prove to be ineffective. So, again, the effectiveness of the therapy, whether psychological or physiological, depends largely on the reasons for the depression.

In summary, the aim of this chapter has been to evaluate some of the more influential psychological treatments for depression. Many limitations are associated with psychological therapies. However, there is a role for both antidepressant drugs and talk therapy in treating depression.

IV

Recommendations for Improving Diagnosis and Treatment

12

Toward an Improvement in Treatment

Throughout this book, I have pointed out some of the many problems currently associated with drug and talk treatments for depression and call for a more uniform approach to theorizing about, diagnosing, and treating the illness.

RECOMMENDED DIAGNOSTIC PROCESS

Because the theoretical considerations have already been presented for discussion, any further exploration would be unnecessarily repetitive. It is helpful just to make a final note that these theoretical reformulations underpin the diagnostic and treatment processes.

The Physician's Role

Before treatments can be prescribed, it is essential that every patient be diagnosed thoroughly to determine if he or she is suffering from primary or secondary depression. To distinguish between primary and secondary depression, the diagnosis should consist of a complete medical evaluation. Even if physicians and therapists are reasonably convinced that their patient's symptoms of depression are caused by a job loss, the breakdown of a marriage, or some other personal catastrophe or major life event, the patient nevertheless should first be medically examined to rule out or to confirm this diagnosis.

This examination should be thorough, and include a complete check on the patient's background to determine major life milestones, current relationships, work, hobbies and interests, and sources of social support and other relevant factors. The medical history should determine existing health problems or illnesses, the onset and development of depressed symptoms, and genetic predisposition to develop the illness by identifying any family members with depression. Medical tests that will verify objectively the information obtained should be included. Blood tests can determine electrolyte imbalances and mineral deficiencies, and diagnostic measures are available to determine whether neurotransmitter levels are abnormal.

Since neuroendocrine problems are often misdiagnosed as depression, they must be ruled out. Physicians can easily evaluate hormone levels to determine whether an imbalance exists. One such test, the *thyroid releasing hormone* (TRH) *stimulation test*, can help determine subclinical hypothyroidism. Because the thyroid gland is linked to the pituitary and the hypothalamus, the TRH stimulation test will reveal any breakdowns in the system. Another neuroendocrine test that should be done is the *dexamethasone suppression test* (DST). Dexamethasone is used to detect excessive levels of cortisol in the system. Both the TRH and DST tests can help identify physiological disturbances in the overwhelming majority of unipolar cases.

Other important tests can be given to determine sleep pattern disturbances. An EEG should show any shortening of REM latency. Brain scans, including magnetic resonance imaging and positron emission topography, may also be useful.

The physician should always ask for information about drug use and abuse, either legal or illegal, whether prescription or over-the-counter, and alcohol consumption.

If these tests all prove negative, a psychiatric or psychological assessment may be necessary.

Restoring Dignity and Respect in Treating Depression

Whatever treatment strategies are prescribed, they are likely to be more effective when health care professionals cease stigmatizing individuals with depression and accept that mood disorders do not result from moral weakness and character flaws. Because depressed patients and clients can require long-term therapy, judgmental attitudes are likely to impede treatment progress and discourage patients from seeking much needed help.

Below are some guidelines for treatment, which I have adapted from the British General Medical Council. These guidelines suggest that health care professionals should:

1. Give the patients or clients information about their condition and communicate in ways that they understand
2. Treat clients and patients politely and with dignity
3. Listen carefully to what they have to say and respect their views
4. Respect their right to take an active involvement in their health care
5. Accept their right to ask for a second opinion
6. Maintain confidentiality and request permission before disclosing details about a client's condition to others
7. Be accessible to the client when on duty

The Patient's Role

While physicians obviously have a central role in diagnosing depression, patients must also be encouraged to take active control of their health management. Although many medical professionals prefer the "good patient," the person who does not challenge the physician, evidence has shown that patients who are involved with their health care are precisely those people who thrive and survive. By contrast, patients who remain passive and surrender control of their health to medical staff are less likely to improve.

One way patients can contribute to their diagnosis is by keeping a diary or journal of their symptoms. When patients document their symptoms on a regular basis in this way, it allows them to discover patterns and trends in their illness and the onset of their symptoms that will provide valuable clues about their illness. Keeping a diary was essential for my client Shelly's recovery.

The process can be time-consuming and laborious, particularly for a depressed person who is likely to have motivational and concentration difficulties. However, they should be encouraged to persevere. Even if the process takes weeks, months, or years, keeping a daily record is important. Clients should include the following various day-to-day items:

- Their overall mental health
- Rate their mental health on a daily basis
- Record all food and alcohol intake
- Chart the weather
- Menstrual cycle, childbirth, and menopause
- Record all prescription and nonprescription drugs
- Make note of the onset of symptoms including the time of day
- Changes in symptoms and the development of any new ones
- Life stressors and disappointments
- Sleeping disturbances
- The effects of exercise and relaxation techniques
- The effects of all medications and psychological treatments
- Note when symptoms disappear

RECOMMENDATIONS FOR TREATMENT

Once the diagnosis is made and, as much as possible, primary or secondary depression is identified, the physician and patient are in a better position to discuss the most appropriate course of treatment. I would advocate both antidepressant treatments and psychological therapy for depressed patients, but it is the individual circumstances in each case that must determine which strategy or strategies to adopt. In some instances, drugs alone might be sufficient, while in others antidepressants combined with therapy might be more beneficial.

While I believe that psychological treatments can benefit the depressed client, I would argue that treatments that are short term and emphasize problem-solving goals are preferable. Although exploring potential childhood causes of the depression may be illuminating, this practice is time-consuming, potentially very traumatic, and unlikely to guarantee a resolution. In my view, psychological treatments, such as cognitive-behavioral and interpersonal therapies, that stress practical strategies to improving the quality of the individual's life, offer support and coping strategies for the effects of this debilitating illness, and provide a program to develop and build self-esteem and confidence are more beneficial. Even if the patient is suffering from secondary depression, its disabling effects can be powerful and frightening and the individual may still need confidence building and support.

Therapies such as humanistic and client-centered approaches should be avoided, because they can increase suffering.

Nontraditional Forms of Treatment

Although traditional forms of treatment, whether medical or psychological, can greatly improve patients' symptoms, other forms of assistance and support can also be beneficial. Therapeutic massage, reflexology, homeopathy, and meditation can all have calming and soothing effects. Relaxation exercises are particularly easy to teach and clients can learn to do them on their own, in between therapy sessions. I would strongly recommend Progressive Relaxation techniques, developed by Edmund Jacobson in the 1930s to alleviate symptoms of anxiety. With this technique, clients are instructed to alternately tense and relax the different muscles in the body. I usually suggest my clients begin with their feet, followed by their calves, thighs, stomach, arms, hands, back, neck, and face.

I am also a great believer in encouraging my clients to keep themselves informed about the latest breakthroughs in and treatments for depression, to join or even start support groups, and to adopt habits leading to an overall sense of physical and emotional well-being.

Because depressed people often feel that their future is futile and hopeless, I advocate countering these negative and destructive views through encouraging goal-setting and personal development. Even after successful therapy, many clients still have to come to terms with the trauma of having suffered depression. Their self-esteem, sense of identity, and views on their life are also often shaky. To help them build confidence and discover new goals, I have designed Rational-Intuitive Therapy, a program of personal development.

Although the general aim of this program is to provide therapeutic assistance for people who need psychological support in a time of transition or personal loss, its focus is on personal development and confidence building through self-reflection and goal formation which also can benefit depressed individuals. The basis principles of Rational-Intuitive Therapy are:

1. To offer clients a choice of treatments. Rational-Intuitive Therapy is a new approach to personal development. It rejects many of the current therapeutic trends, particularly those that focus on the need for the client to first deal with the past in order to face the future. This insistence on rooting around in someone's past is not only often unnecessarily painful and traumatic for the client, but it also cannot guarantee that this insight will lead to any improvement.

   The Rational-Intuitive approach, in contrast, is much more positive, dynamic, and forward looking. Irrespective of one's childhood, everyone has within them the potential for improvement and fulfillment and the therapist and client must start with the present and look forward.

2. To provide an atmosphere for personal exploration, self-awareness, and personal development that is supportive and respectful of the client and his or her needs. The therapist's role is to help individuals rediscover goals, to foster confidence and bolster self-esteem.

3. To provide practical solutions that will help people define and achieve goals, make improvements and changes, create new opportunities, and ultimately lead to personal fulfillment and satisfaction.

4. Most importantly, to encourage the client that changes and improvements, happiness and personal fulfillment are possible. Sometimes people, particularly those who are depressed, are convinced that they are not worthy of success and happiness. This negative mind-set, unfortunately, influences the way people live and think about themselves. The Rational-Intuitive approach to personal development helps people overcome their negative thoughts and belief systems.

These recommendations represent some of the more fundamental and necessary ways to improve diagnosis and treatment. However, the list is by no means exhaustive. As a result, I have most likely introduced many more questions into the diagnostic and treatment processes than I have provided answers for. This undoubtedly reflects the nature of researching a complex disease like depression.

In summing up, it is to be stressed that mood disorders are much more complicated illnesses than many current forms of diagnosis and treatment would suggest. No two cases of depression are alike, whether in the origins of the symptoms or the way in which they respond to treatment. Health care professionals must continue to explore a wide range of potential causes, be flexible with treatments, and encourage their patients to take an active involvement in their health care. Together, as a team, the practitioner and patient can work to ensure the best forms of treatment possible.

References

Abramson *et al.* (1978). Learned helplessness in humans: Critique and reformulation. *Journal of Abnormal Psychology, 87,* 49–74.

Abramson *et al.* (1989). Hopelessness depression: A theory based sub-type of depression. *Psychological Review, 96,* 358–372.

Akiskal, Hagop. (1990). *Dysthymic disorder.* New York: Gaskell.

Alloy, Lauren. (1988). *Cognitive processes in depression.* New York: Guilford Press.

American Psychological Association. (1994). *Diagnostic and statistical manual of mental disorders* (4th ed.). Washington, DC: Author.

Beck, Aaron. (1967). *Depression: Causes and treatment.* Philadelphia: University of Pennsylvania Press.

Beck, Aaron. (1980). *Cognitive therapy for depression.* New York: Wiley.

Billig, Nathan. (1987). *Too old and sad: Understanding depression in the elderly.* Lexington, MA: Lexington Books.

Bowlby, John. (1973). *Separation and loss.* New York: Basic Books.

Brewin, C. R. (1985). Depression and causal attributes: What is their relation? *Psychological Bulletin, 98,* 297–307.

Brown, George. (1979). *Social origins of depression: A study of psychiatric disorder in women.* London: Tavistock.

Carlson, N. (1986). *Physiology of behavior* (3rd ed.). Boston: Allyn & Bacon.

Chester, Rosie. (1995). *Older people's sadness.* London: Counsel and Care.

Cialdini, Robert B. (1982). *Influence: How and why people agree to things.* New York: Quill.

Costello, Charles. (1993). *Symptoms of depression.* New York: Wiley.

Coyne, J. C., & Gotlieb, I. H. (1983). The role of cognition in depression: A critical appraisal. *Psychological Bulletin, 94,* 472–505.

Davidson, R. J. (1992). Emotion and affective style. Hemispheric substrates. *Psychological Science, 3*, 39–43.

Downing-Orr, K. (1996). *Alienation and social support: A social psychological study of homeless young people in London and in Sydney*. Aldershot, England: Avebury Press.

Eaton, W. W., Kramer, M., Anthony, J. C., Dryman, A., & Shapiro, S. (1989). The incidence of specific DIS/DSM-III mental disorders: Data from the NIMH Epidemiologic Catchment Area programs. *Acta Psychiatrica Scandinavica, 79*, 163–178.

Egeland, J. A., Gerhard, D. S., Pauls, D. L., Sussex, J. W., Kidd, K. K., Allen, C. R., Hostetter, A. M., & Houseman, D. E. (1987). Bipolar affective disorders linked to DNA markers on chromosome 11. *Nature, 325*, 783–787.

Ellis, Albert. (1962). *Reason and emotion in psychotherapy*. Secaucus, NJ: Lyle Stuart.

European College of Neuropsychopharmacology. (1995). *8th International Psychiatric Conference*, Venice, Italy.

Ferster, Charles. (1975). *Behavior principles*. Englewood Cliffs, NJ: Prentice–Hall.

Gold, Mark. (1995). *The good news about depression*. New York: Fireside Books.

Goodwin, F. K., Wir-Justice, A., & Wehr, T. A. (1982). Affective disorders caused by disturbance in circadian rhythms. In E. Costa & G. Ralagni (Eds.), *Typical and atypical anti-depressants: Clinical practice* (pp. 142–165) New York: Raven.

Gotlib, Ian, & Hammen, Constance. (1992). *Psychological aspects of depression*. New York: Wiley.

Gut, Emmy. (1988). *Productive and unproductive depression: Success or failure of a vital process*. London: Tavistock/Routledge.

Klein, M. (1935). A contribution to the psychogenesis of manic-depressive states. In *The Writings of Melanie Klein* (vol. 1, pp. 262–289). London, Hogarth.

Levanthal, H. (1980). Towards a comprehensive theory of emotion. *Advances in Experimental Social Psychology, 13*, 139–207.

Lewinsohn, Peter. (1978). *Control your depression*. Englewood Cliffs, NJ: Prentice–Hall.

Mendlewicz, J., & Montgomery, S. A. (1995). *Mirtazepine: A noradrengic and specific serotonergic antidepressant* (Proceedings of a satellite symposium of the VIIIth Congress of the European College of Neuropsychopharmacology). London: Rapid Science.

Milligan, S., & Clare, A. (1994). *Depression and how to survive it*. London: Ebury.

Nolen-Hoeksema, S. (1987). Sex differences in unipolar depression: Evidence and theory. *Psychological Bulletin, 101*, 259–282.

Orley, J. (1970). *Culture and mental illness: A study from Uganda*. Nairobi: E. African Publishing House.

Payer, Lynn. (1988). *Medicine and culture: Varieties of treatment in the United States, England, West Germany, and France*. New York: Penguin.

Paykel, E. S. (1979). *Psychopharmacology of affective disorders*. New York: Oxford University Press.

Plath, Sylvia. (1963). *The bell jar*. London: Faber & Faber.

Rosenthal *et al.* (1988). Phototherapy for seasonal affective disorder: A description of syndrome and preliminary findings with light therapy. *Archives of General Psychiatry, 41*, 72–80.

Schuyler, D. (1974). *The depression spectrum*. New York: Aronson.

Seligman, M. E. P. (1989a). Research in clinical psychology: Why is there so much depression today? In I. S. Cohen (Ed.), *The G. Stanley Hall lecture series* (vol. 9, pp. 75–96). Washington, DC: American Psychological Association.

Seligman, Martin. (1989b). *Helplessness: On depression, development and death*. San Francisco: Freeman.

Wilhelm, K., & Parker, G. (1989). Is sex necessarily a risk factor to depression? *Psychological Medicine, 18*, 401–413.

Bibliography

Bartholini, Giuseppe. (1986). *GABA and mood disorders*. New York: Raven Press.

Becker, Robert. (1987). *Social skills training for depression*. Elmsford, NY: Pergamon Press.

Davis, J. M. (1985). Anti-depressant drugs. In H. I. Kaplan & T. Sadock (Eds.), *Comprehensive textbook of psychiatry* (4th ed., p. 300). Baltimore: Williams & Wilkins.

Dean, Alfred. (1986). *Social support, life events and depression*. New York: Academic Press.

Depue, Richard. (1979). *The psychobiology of depressive disorders*. New York: Academic Press.

Ellis, A., & Dryden, W. (1987). *The practice of rational emotive therapy*. Berlin: Springer.

Gilbert, Paul. (1984). *Depression: From psychology to brain state*. Hillsdale, NJ: Erlbaum.

Gilbert, Paul. (1992). *Depression: The evolution of powerlessness*. Hillsdale, NJ: Erlbaum.

Gotlib, Ian, & Colby, Catherine. (1987). *Treatment of depression: An interpersonal systems approach*. Elmsford, NY: Pergamon Press.

Horton, R. W. (1994). *Biological aspects of affective disorders*. New York: Karge.

Marsella, Anthony, Hirshfeld, R. M., & Katz, M. (1987). *The measurement of depression*. New York: Wiley.

Petty, Richard. (1987). *Depression: Treating the whole person*. New York: Unwin Paperbacks.

Robbins, Paul. (1993). *Understanding depression*. London: McFarland.

Rowe, Dorothy. (1983). *Depression: The way out of your prison*. London: Routledge.

Rowe, Dorothy. (1991). *Breaking the bonds: Understanding depression, finding freedom*. London: Fontana.

Sadock, B., & Kaplan, I. (1995). *Comprehensive textbook of psychiatry*. Baltimore: Williams & Wilkins.

Schatzberg, Alan. (1988). *The hypothalamic–pituitary–adrenal axis: Physiology, pathophysiology, and psychiatry implications*. New York: Raven Press.

Shapiro, Colin. (1994). Sleep disorders in anxiety and depression. *Journal of Psychosomatic Research, 38*, 125–139.

Williams, J., & Mark, G. (1984). *The psychological treatment of depression*. London: Croom Helm.

Willmer, Paul. (1985). *Depression: A psychobiological synthesis*. New York: Wiley.

Index